Virtual Clinical Excursi

for

Phipps, Monahan, Sands, Marek, and Neighbors

MEDICAL-SURGICAL NURSING:
Health and Illness Perspectives
7th Edition

Virtual Clinical Excursions

for

Phipps, Monahan, Sands, Marek, and Neighbors

MEDICAL-SURGICAL NURSING:
Health and Illness Perspectives
7th Edition

prepared by

Mary Ann Hogan, RN, CS, MSN
Clinical Assistant Professor
School of Nursing
University of Massachusetts
Amherst, Massachusetts

Virtual Clinical Excursions CD-ROM prepared by

Jay Shiro Tashiro, PhD, RN
Director of Systems Design
Wolfsong Informatics
Tucson, Arizona

Gina Long, RN, DNSc
Assistant Professor, Department of Nursing
College of Health Professions
Northern Arizona University
Flagstaff, Arizona

Ellen Sullins, PhD
Director of Research
Wolfsong Informatics
Tucson, Arizona

Michael Kelly, MS
Director of the Center for Research and
Evaluation of Advanced Technologies
in Education
Northern Arizona University
Flagstaff, Arizona

The development of *Virtual Clinical Excursions* Volume 1 was partially funded by the
National Science Foundation, under grant DUE 9950613.
Principal investigators were Tashiro, Sullins, Long, and Kelly.

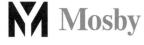 Mosby

An Imprint of Elsevier Science
St. Louis   London   Philadelphia   Sydney   Toronto

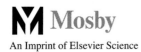 **Mosby**

An Imprint of Elsevier Science

11830 Westline Industrial Drive
St. Louis, Missouri 63146

Virtual Clinical Excursions for Phipps, Monahan, Sands, Marek, and Neighbors: ISBN 0-323-02338-x
Medical-Surgical Nursing: Health and Illness Perspectives, 7th edition
Copyright © 2003,   Mosby, Inc.   All rights reserved.

Notice

Pharmacology is an ever-changing field. Standard safety precautions must be followed, but as new research
and clinical experience broaden our knowledge, changes in treatment and drug therapy may become necessary or appropriate. Readers are advised to check the most current product information provided by the
manufacturer of each drug to be administered to verify the recommended dose, the method and duration of
administration, and contraindications. It is the responsibility of the licensed prescriber, relying on experience and knowledge of the patient, to determine dosages and the best treatment for each individual patient.
Neither the publisher nor the editor assumes any liability for any injury and/or damage to persons or prop-
erty arising from this publication.

The Publisher

First Edition 2003.

Vice President and Publishing Director, Nursing: Sally Schrefer
Acquisitions Editor: Tom Wilhelm
Senior Developmental Editor: Jeff Downing
Project Manager: Gayle Morris
Designer: Wordbench
Cover Art: Kathi Gosche

WB/MVB

Printed in the United States of America

Last digit is the print number: 9   8   7   6   5   4   3   2   1

Workbook
prepared by

Mary Ann Hogan, RN, CS, MSN
Clinical Assistant Professor
School of Nursing
University of Massachusetts
Amherst, Massachusetts

Textbook

Wilma J. Phipps, PhD, RN, FAAN
Professor Emeritus of Medical-Surgical Nursing
Frances Payne Bolton School of Nursing
Case Western Reserve University
Cleveland, Ohio

Frances D. Monahan, PhD, RN
Professor and Director
Department of Nursing
Rockland Community College
State University of New York
Suffern, New York

Judith K. Sands, RN, EdD
Associate Professor
School of Nursing
University of Virginia
Charlottesville, Virginia

Jane F. Marek, MSN, RN, CS
Adult Nurse Practitioner
Instructor
Frances Payne Bolton School of Nursing
Case Western Reserve University
Cleveland, Ohio

Marianne Neighbors, EdD, RN
Professor
School of Nursing
University of Arkansas
Fayetteville, Arkansas

Contents

Part VIII—Neurologic Problems

Part IX—Musculoskeletal Problems

Part X—Immunologic Problems

Part XI—Skin Problems

Getting Started

GETTING SET UP

■ MINIMUM SYSTEM REQUIREMENTS

Virtual Clinical Excursions is a hybrid CD, so it runs on both Macintosh and Windows platforms. To use *Virtual Clinical Excursions*, you will need one of the following systems:

- **Windows™**

  Windows 2000, 95, 98, NT 4.0
  IBM compatible computer
  Pentium II processor (or equivalent)
  300 MHz
  96 MB
  800 × 600 screen size
  256 color monitor
  100 MB hard drive space
  12× CD-ROM drive
  Soundblaster 16 soundcard compatibility
  Stereo speakers or headphones

- **Macintosh®**

  MAC OS 9.04
  Apple Power PC G3
  300 MHz
  96 MB
  800 × 600 screen size
  256 color monitor
  100 MB hard drive space
  12× CD-ROM drive
  Stereo speakers or headphones

Ideally, the system you use should have at least 200 MB of free disk space on your hard drive. There are commercially available desktop utility programs that can help clean up your hard drive. No other applications besides the operating system should be running at the time *Virtual Clinical Excursions* is running.

1

■ INSTALLING *VIRTUAL CLINICAL EXCURSIONS*

Virtual Clinical Excursions is designed to run from a set of files on your hard drive and a CD in your CD-ROM. Minimal installation is required.

- **Windows™**

    1. Start Microsoft Windows and insert *Virtual Clinical Excursions* **Disk 1 (Installation)** in the CD-ROM drive.
    2. Click the **Start** icon on the taskbar and select the **Run** option.
    3. Type d:\setup.exe (where "d:\" is your CD-ROM drive) and press OK.
    4. Follow the on-screen instructions for installation.
    5. Remove *Virtual Clinical Excursions* **Disk 1 (Installation)** from your CD-ROM drive.
    6. Restart your computer.

- **Macintosh®**

    1. Insert *Virtual Clinical Excursions* **Disk 1 (Installation)** in the CD-ROM drive. The disk icon will appear on your desktop.
    2. Double-click on the disk icon.
    3. Double-click on the icon **Install Virtual Clinical Excursions**.
    4. Follow the on-screen instructions for installation.
    5. Remove *Virtual Clinical Excursions* **Disk 1 (Installation)** from your CD-ROM drive
    6. Restart your computer.

■ HOW TO RESET YOUR MONITOR TO 256 COLORS

This software will only run if the monitor is set at 256 colors. To reset your monitor:

- **Windows™**

    1. Choose **Settings** from the **Start** menu.
    2. Choose **Control Panel**.
    3. Double-click on the **Display** icon.
    4. Click on the **Settings** tab.
    5. In the **Colors** drop-down menu, click on the arrow to show more settings.
    6. Click on **256 Colors**.
    7. Click on **Apply**.
    8. Click on **OK**.
    9. If the system asks whether you wish to restart your computer to accept these settings, click on **Yes**.

- **Macintosh®**

    1. Choose the **Monitors** control panel.
    2. Change the color display to **256**.

■ HOW TO USE DISK 2 (PATIENTS' DISK)

- **Windows™**

  When you want to work with the five patients in the virtual hospital, follow these steps:

  1. Insert *Virtual Clinical Excursions* **Disk 2 (Patients' Disk)** into your CD-ROM drive.
  2. Double-click on the icon **Shortcut to Virtual Clinical Excursions**, which can be found on your desktop. This will load and run the program.

- **Macintosh®**

  When you want to work with the five patients in the virtual hospital, follow these steps:

  1. Insert *Virtual Clinical Excursions* **Disk 2 (Patients' Disk)** into your CD-ROM drive.
  2. Double-click on the icon **Shortcut to Virtual Clinical Excursions**, which can be found on your desktop. This will load and run the program.

■ QUALITY OF VISUALS, SPEED, AND COMMON PROBLEMS

Virtual Clinical Excursions uses the Apple QuickTime media layer system. This includes Quick-Time Video and QuickTime VR Video, which allow for high-quality graphics and digital video. The graphics seen in the *Virtual Clinical Excursions* courseware should be of high quality with good color. If the movies and graphics appear blocky or otherwise low-quality, check to see whether your video card is set to "thousands of colors."

Note: Virtual Clinical Excursions is not designed to function at a 256-color depth. (You may need to go to the Control Panel and change the Display settings.) If you don't see any digital video options, please check that QuickTime is installed correctly.

The system should respond quickly and smoothly. In particular, you should not see any jerky motions or unannounced long delays as you move through the virtual hospital settings, interact with patients, or access information resources. If you notice slow, jerky, or delayed software responses, it may mean that your particular system requires additional RAM, your processor does not meet the basic requirements, or your hard drive is full or too fragmented. If the videos appear banded or subject to "breakup," you may need to find an updated video driver for the computer's video card. Please consult the manufacturer of the video card or computer for additional video drivers for your machine.

■ TECHNICAL SUPPORT

Technical support for this product is available at no charge by calling the Technical Support Hotline between 9 a.m. and 5 p.m. (Central Time), Monday through Friday. Inside the United States, call 1-800-692-9010. Outside the United States, call 314-872-8370.

A QUICK TOUR

Welcome to *Virtual Clinical Excursions*, a virtual hospital setting in which you can work with five complex patient simulations and also learn to access and evaluate the information resources that are essential for high-quality patient care.

The virtual hospital, Red Rock Canyon Medical Center, is a teaching hospital for Canyonlands State University. Within the medical center, you will work on a medical-surgical floor with a realistic architecture as well as access information resources. The floor plan in which the patient scenarios unfold is constructed from a model of a real medical center. The medical-surgical unit has:

- Five patient rooms (Room 302, Room 303, Room 304, Room 309, Room 310)
- A Nurses' Station (Room 312)
- A Supervisor's Office (Room 301)
- Two conference rooms (Room 307, Room 308)
- A nurses' lounge (Room 306)

■ BEFORE YOU START

Make sure you have your textbook nearby when you use the *Virtual Clinical Excursions Patients' Disk*. You will want to consult topic areas in your textbook frequently while working with the CD and using this workbook.

■ SUPERVISOR'S OFFICE (ROOM 301)

Just like a real-world clinical rotation, you have to let someone know when you arrive on the hospital floor—and you have to let someone know when you leave the floor. This process is completed in the Supervisor's Office (Room 301).

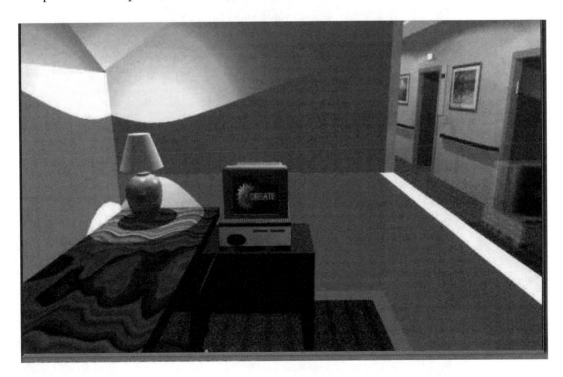

To get a 360° view of where you are "standing":

- Place the cursor in the middle of the screen.
- Hold down the mouse.
- Drag either right or left.

You will see you are in a room with an alcove to your left and a door behind you. To move into the hallway, place the cursor in the door opening and click. Once you are in the hallway, hold down the mouse and make a 360° turn.

In one direction, you will see:

- An exit sign
- An elevator
- A waiting room

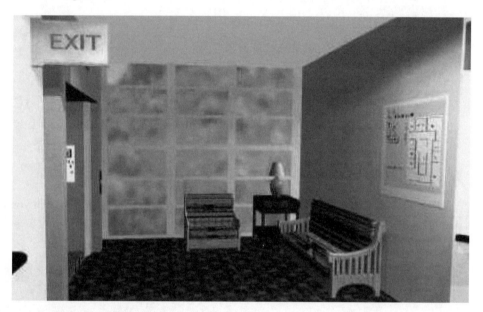

In the other direction, you will see a:

- Patient room
- Mobile computer

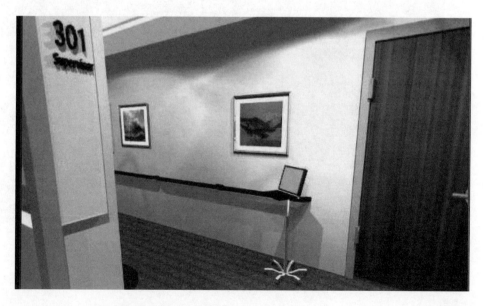

Move the cursor to a new place along the hallway outside the Supervisor's Office and click again. (Always try to place the cursor in the middle of the screen.) You should be moving along the hallway. Remember, at any point you can hold down the mouse and turn 360° in either direction. You can also hold down and move the mouse to the top or bottom of the frame, giving you views looking up or down.

■ READING ROOM

Go back into the Supervisor's Office by clicking on anything inside the room. Explore the Supervisor's Office (Room 301), and you will find another computer. This computer is a link to Canyonlands State University, the simulated university associated with the Red Rock Canyon Medical Center. Double-click on this computer, and a Web browser screen will be launched, which will open the Medical-Nursing Library in Canyonlands State University.

Click on the **Reading Room** icon, and you will see a table of icons that allows you to read short learning modules on a variety of anatomy and physiology topics.

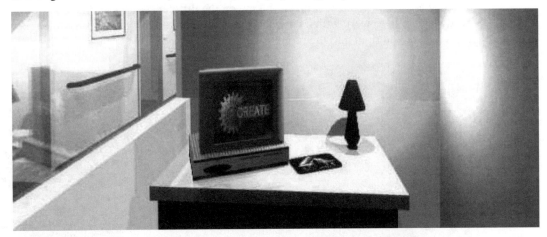

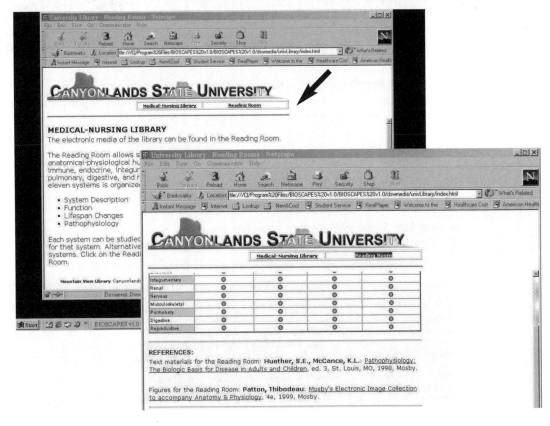

When you are ready to exit the reading room, go to the **File** icon on the browser, look at the drop-down menu, and select **Exit** or **Close**, depending on your Web browser. The browser will close, and once again you will be looking at the computer in the Supervisor's Office.

■ FLOOR MAP AND ANIMATED MAP

Move into the hallway outside the Supervisor's Office and turn right. A floor map can be found on the wall in the waiting area opposite the elevator and exit sign. To get there, click on anything in the waiting area. You should be able to see the map now, but you may not be close enough to open it. Click again on an object in the waiting area; this will move you closer. Turn to the right until you can see the map. Double-click on the map, and you will get a close-up view of the medical-surgical floor's layout. Click on the **Return** icon to exit this close-up view of the floor map.

Compare the floor map on the wall with the animated map in the upper right-hand corner of your screen. The green dot follows your position on the floor to show you where you are. You can move about the floor by double-clicking on the different rooms in this map. If you have already signed in to work with a patient, double-clicking on the patient's room on the animated map will take you right into the room.

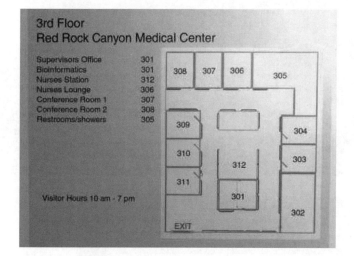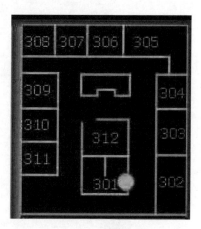

Note: If you have not signed in to work with a patient, double-clicking on a patient's room on the animated map will take you to the hallway right outside the room. If you have not yet selected a patient, you cannot access patient rooms or records.

■ HOW TO SIGN IN

To select a patient, you will need to sign in on the desktop computer in the Supervisor's Office (Room 301). Double-click on the computer screen, and a log-on screen will appear.

- Replace *Student Name* with your name.
- Replace the student ID number with your student ID number.
- Click **Continue** in the lower right side of the screen.

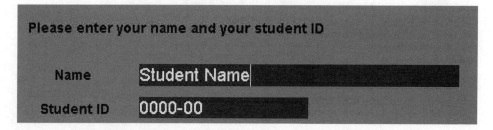

■ HOW TO SELECT A PATIENT

You can choose any one of five patients to work with. For each patient you can select either of two 4-hour shifts on Tuesday or Thursday (0700–1100 or 1100–1500). You can also select a Friday morning period in which you can review all of the data for the patient you selected. You will not, however, be able to visit patients on Friday, only review their records.

■ PATIENT LIST

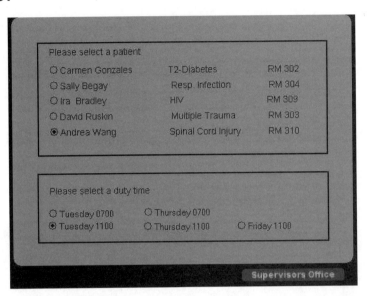

- **Carmen Gonzales (Room 302)**

  Diabetes mellitus, type 2 – An older Hispanic female with an infected leg that has become gangrenous. She has type 2 diabetes mellitus, as well as complications of congestive heart failure and osteomyelitis.

- **David Ruskin (Room 303)**

  Motor vehicle accident – A young adult African-American male admitted with a possible closed head injury and a severely fractured right humerus following a car-bicycle accident. He undergoes an open reduction and internal fixations of the right humerus.

- **Sally Begay (Room 304)**

  Respiratory infection – A Native American woman initially suspected to have a Hantavirus infection. She has a confirmed diagnosis of bacterial lung infection. This patient's complications include chronic obstructive pulmonary disease and inactive tuberculosis.

- **Ira Bradley (Room 309)**

  HIV-AIDS – A Caucasian adult male in late-stage HIV infection admitted for an opportunistic respiratory infection. He has complications of oral fungal infection, malnutrition, and wasting. Patient-family interactions also provide opportunities to explore complex psychosocial problems.

- **Andrea Wang (Room 310)**

  Spinal cord injury – A young Asian female who entered the hospital after a diving accident in which her T6 was crushed, with partial transection of the spinal cord. After a week in ICU, she has been transferred to the Medical-Surgical unit, where she is being closely monitored.

Note: You can select only one patient for one time period. If you are assigned to work with multiple patients, return to the Supervisor's Office to switch from one patient to another.

■ HOW TO FIND A PATIENT'S RECORDS

Nurses' Station (Room 312)

Within the Nurses' Station, you will see:

1. A blue notebook on the counter—this is the Medication Administration Record (MAR).
2. A bookshelf with patient charts.
3. Two desktop computers—the computer to the left of the bulletin board is used to access Red Rock Canyon Medical Center's Intranet; the computer to the right beneath the bookshelf is used to access the Electronic Patient Record (EPR). *(Note: You can also access the EPR from the mobile computer outside the Supervisor's Office, next to Room 302.)*
4. A bulletin board—this contains important information for students.

As you use these resources, you will always be able to return to the Nurses' Station (Room 312) by clicking either a **Nurses' Station** icon or a **3rd Floor** icon located next to the red cross in the lower right-hand corner of the computer screen.

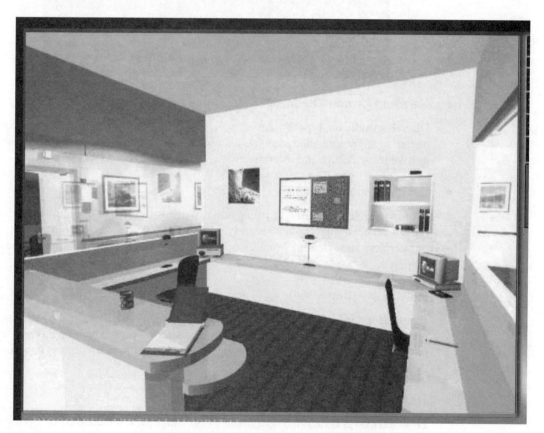

1. Medication Administration Record (MAR)

The blue notebook on the counter in the Nurses' Station (Room 312) is the Medication Adminis-tration Record (MAR), listing current 24-hour medications for each patient. Simply click on the MAR, and it opens like a notebook. Tabs allow you to select patients by room number. Each MAR sheet lists the following:

- Medications
- Route and dosage of medications
- Times of administration of medication

The MAR changes each day.

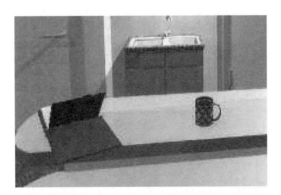

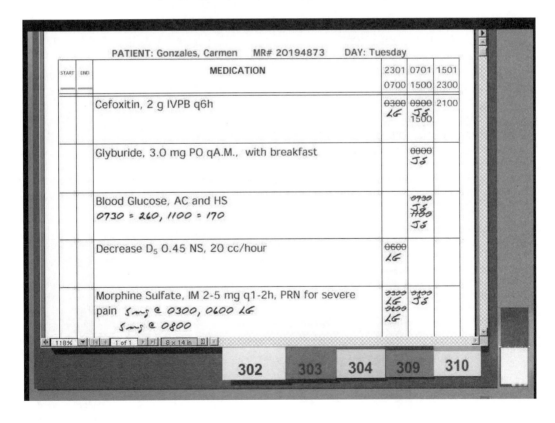

2. Charts

In the back right-hand corner of the Nurses' Station (Room 312) is a bookshelf with patient charts. To open a chart:

- Double-click on the bookshelf.
- Click once on the chart of your choice.

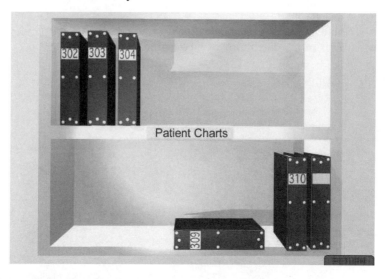

Tabs at the bottom of each patient's chart allow you to review the following data:

- Physical History*
- Physicians' Notes
- Physicians' Orders
- Nurses' Notes
- Diagnostics Reports

- Expired MARs
- Health Team Reports
- Surgeons' Notes
- Other Reports

"Flip" forward by selecting a tab or backward by clicking on the small chart icon in the lower right side of your screen. (**Flip Back** appears on this icon once you have moved beyond the first tab.) As in the real world, the data in each patient's chart changes daily.

Note: The Physical History tab of the chart contains the patient's History and Physical data and, for some patients, the Emergency Department Record. Remember to scroll down to read all pages.

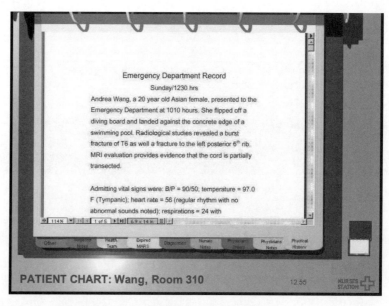

3. Two Computers

◆   **Electronic Patient Record (EPR)**

You can access an Electronic Patient Record (EPR) only after you have signed in and selected the patient in the Supervisor's Office (Room 301). The EPR can be accessed from two computers:

- Desktop computer under the bookshelf in the Nurses' Station (Room 312)
- Mobile computer outside the Supervisor's Office, next to Room 302

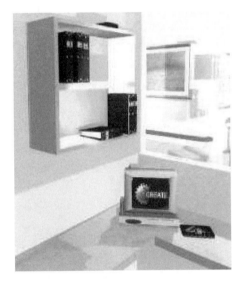
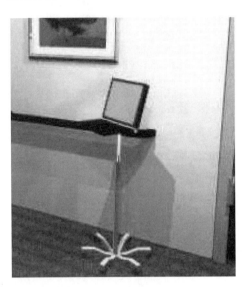

To access a patient's EPR:

- Double-click on the computer screen.
- Type in the password—it will always be **rn2b**.
- Click on **Access Records**.
- Click on the patient's name, then on **Access EPR** (or simply double-click on the patient's name).

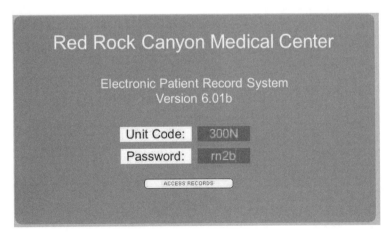

Note: Do **not** *press the Return/Enter key. If you make a mistake, simply delete the password, reenter it, and click* **Access Records**. *You will then enter the records system, where you find a list of patients.*

The EPR form represents a composite of commercial versions being used in hospitals and clinics. You can access the EPR:

- For a patient
- To review existing data
- To enter data you collect while working with a patient

The EPR is updated daily, so no matter what day or part of a shift you are working, there will be a current EPR with the patient's data from the past days of the current hospital stay. This type of simulated EPR allows you to examine how data for different attributes have changed over time, as well as to examine data for all of a patient's attributes at a particular time. The EPR is fully functional (as it is in a real-life hospital or clinic). You can enter such data as blood pressure, heart rate, and temperature. The EPR will not, however, allow you to enter data for a previous time period.

At the lower left corner of the EPR, there are nine icons that allow you to view different types of patient data:

- Assessment
- Admissions
- Urinanalysis
- Vital Signs
- ADL

- Blood Gases
- I&O
- Chemistry
- Hematology

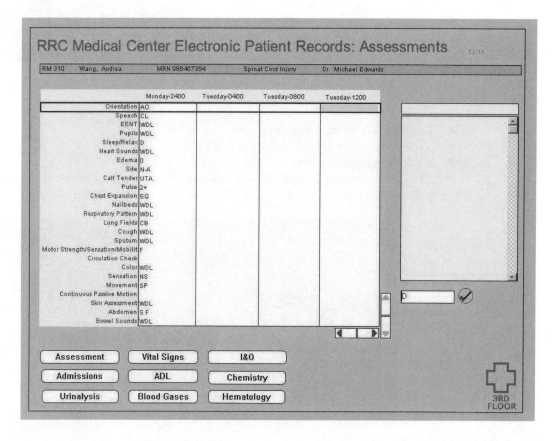

Remember, each hospital or clinic selects its own codes. The codes in the Red Rock Canyon Medical Center may be different from ones you have seen in clinical rotations that have computerized patient records.

You use the codes for the data type, selecting the code to describe your assessment findings and typing that code in the box in the lower right side of the screen, to the left of the checkmark symbol (✓).

Once the data are typed in this box, they are entered into the patient's record by clicking on the checkmark (✓). Make sure you are in the correct cell by looking for the placement of the blue box in the table. That box identifies which cell the database is "looking" at for any given moment.

You can leave the EPR by clicking on the **3rd Floor** icon in the lower right corner. This takes you back into the Nurses' Station (Room 312).

◆ Intranet

The computer on the left of the bulletin board in the Nurses' Station (Room 312) is dedicated to Red Rock Canyon Medical Center's **Intranet**. This system contains resources related to working within the hospital. Again, a double click on the screen will activate the computer. A Web browser will come up with four options (Hospital News, Employment, InfoStat, and Home). Navigate within the Intranet just as you would within a Web-based Internet site. Click on **Hospital News** and read some of the articles. The Employment icon opens a screen with descriptions of jobs available in the hospital. The InfoStat icon will connect the hospital Intranet to the Internet. *(Note: This option searches for your Internet connection, activates that connection, and takes you to the publisher's Website for your textbook.)* When in doubt, click on **Home**, which will take you back to the home page for the site.

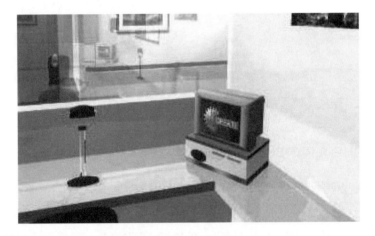

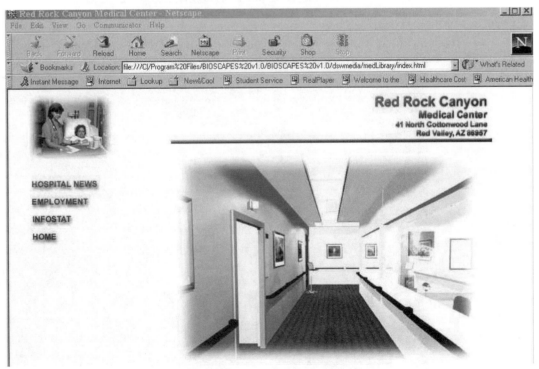

To return to the **Nurses' Station (Room 312)**, exit from the browser. This computer simulates being in a Web environment, so you have to exit from the Intranet by exiting from the browser. Click on **File**, then on **Exit** or **Close** (depending on your browser).

4. Bulletin Board

The bulletin board in the Nurses' Station (Room 312) has important information for students. Click on the board and you can read where reports are being given for patients and where the health team meetings are being held. Lessons in your workbook will direct you to these meetings and reports. Click on **Return** to exit this close-up view of the board.

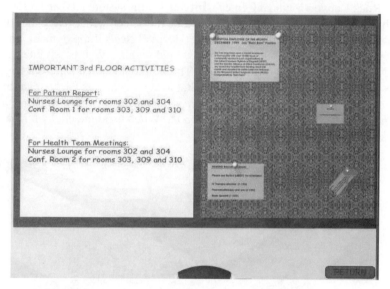

■ VISITING A PATIENT

First, go the Supervisor's Office and sign in to work with Andrea Wang for Tuesday at 0700. Now go to her room. *(Note: The quickest way to get to a patient's room is by double-clicking the room number on the animated map. You can also choose to move through the hallway until you reach the patient's door; then click on the doorknob.)* Once you are inside the room, you will see a still frame of your patient. Below this frame, you will find four icons:

- Vital Signs   • Health History   • Physical   • Medications

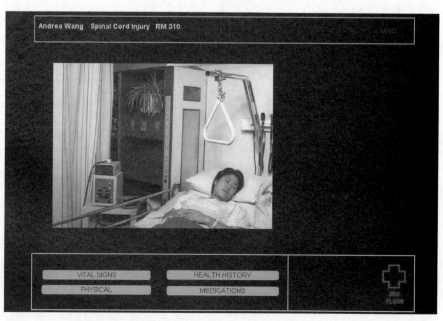

Each of these icons provides the opportunity to assess the patient or the patient's medications. When you click on an icon, you will follow a nurse through the process of collecting assessment data. The nurse will not speak to you but will rely on you to collect the data obtained during patient assessment, to record patient data in the EPR, and sometimes to make decisions after a nurse-patient interaction.

◆   **Vital Signs**

Click on **Vital Signs**; six new icons appear. Each of these new icons allows you to collect data for a particular vital sign. *(Note: You can also see two icons in the right corner. Continue Working with Patient takes you back to the main menu for this patient. Clicking on 3rd Floor will take you back into the hallway.)* Click on the **Temperature** icon. You will see the nurse take the patient's temperature with a tympanic thermometer. At the end of the measurement, the temperature is shown in the animation of the thermometer to the right of the video screen. These types of interactions allow you to collect data during patient visits.

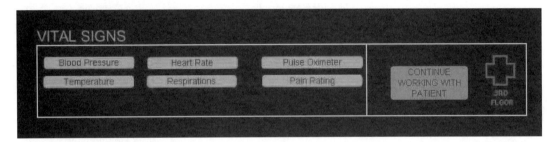

◆   **Physical Examination**

Click **Continue Working with Patient** to return to the main patient menu. Now click the **Physical** icon. Note the different areas of physical examination you can conduct. Try one.

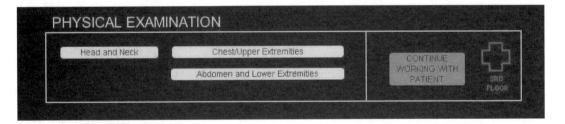

◆   **Health History**

Next, click **Continue Working with Patient** and select the **Health History** icon. In this interactive learning arena, you can ask the patient about her health history. Questions are organized into 12 categories, each of which is accessed by an icon below the video screen. Click on **Culture**, and three new icons appear in the frame to the right of the video. Click on the **Preferred Language** icon, and you will discover the language this patient prefers to use. For each of the 12 question areas, there are three topics you can explore. Thus, there are 36 different question areas related to the health history of each patient.

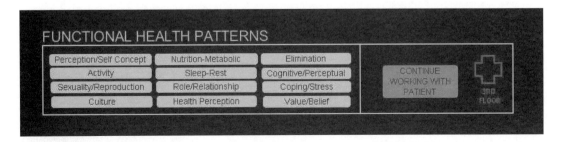

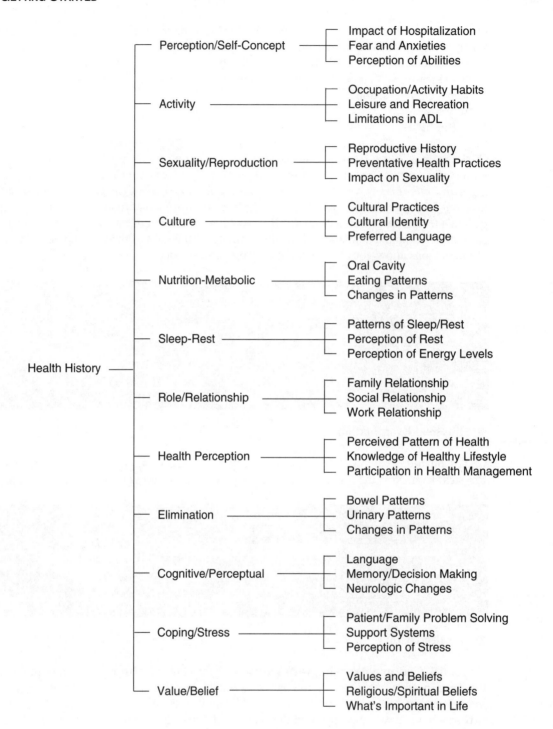

◆   **Medications**

Click **Continue Working with Patient**, and then click the **Medications** icon. Notice that you have three options within this learning environment: Review Medications, Administer, and Hold Medications. Don't click on these now, because you will need to look at this patient's records before you decide whether or not to give medications.

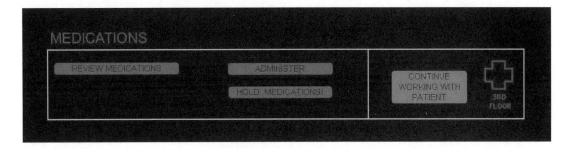

■ HOW TO QUIT OR CHANGE PATIENTS

How to Quit: If necessary, click either the **3rd Floor** icon or the **Nurses' Station** icon (depending on which screen you are currently using) to return to the medical-surgical floor. Then click on the **Quit** icon in the lower right corner of your screen.

How to Change Patients or Shifts: Go to the Supervisor's Office and double-click on the sign-in computer. Click the **Reset** icon. When the next screen appears, select a new patient or a different shift with the same patient.

A DETAILED TOUR

If you wish to understand the capabilities of the virtual hospital, take a detailed tour by going through the following section.

◼ WORKING WITH A PATIENT

Sign in and select Carmen Gonzales as your patient for Tuesday at 0700 hours.

To become more familiar with the *Virtual Clinical Excursions Patients' Disk,* try the following exercises. These activities are designed to introduce you to all of the different components and learning opportunities available within the software. Each exercise will ask you to collect data on a patient.

◼ REPORT

In hospitals, when one nurse's shift ends and another begins, the outgoing nurse who attended a patient will give a verbal and sometimes a written summary of that patient's condition to the incoming nurse who will assume care for the patient. This summary is called a *report* and is an important source of data to provide an overview of a patient.

Your first task is to get the report on Carmen Gonzales. Go to the bulletin board in the Nurses' Station. Double-click on the board and check the location where the attending nurse from the previous shift will give you report on this patient. Remember, Carmen Gonzales is in Room 302, so look for that room number on the bulletin board. You will find that the report is being given in the Nurses' Lounge (Room 306). Click **Return** to leave this close-up view of the bulletin board. *(Note: You can also find out where reports are being given by moving your cursor across the animated map.)* Go to Room 306 by double-clicking on the animated map. Once inside the room, click on **Report** and then on **Gonzales**. Listen to report and make a list of this patient's problems and high-priority concerns. When you are finished, click on the **3rd Floor** icon to return to the Nurses' Station.

Problems/Concerns

■ CHARTS

Find the patient charts in the bookshelf to the right of the bulletin board. Double-click on the bookshelf and find Carmen Gonzales' chart (the one labeled **302**). Click on her chart and read the section called Physical & History, including the Emergency Department Record. Determine from this information why Carmen Gonzales has been admitted to the hospital. In the space below, write a brief summary of why this patient was admitted.

■ MEDICATIONS

Open the Medication Administration Record (MAR) by clicking on the blue notebook on the counter of the Nurses' Station. Find the list of medications prescribed for Carmen Gonzales, and write down the medications that need to be given during the time period 0730–0930. For each medication, note dosage, route, and time in the chart below.

Time	Medication	Dosage	Route

Close the MAR and go inside Carmen Gonzales' room (302). Click on the **Medications** icon. You will be responsible for administering the medications ordered during the time period 0730–0930.

To become familiar with the medication options, look at the frame below the video screen. There you will find three opportunities:

- Review Medications
- Administer
- Hold Medications

Click on **Review Medications**. This brings up a frame to the right of the video screen with a list of the medications ordered for the period 0730–0930 hours. Decide whether these medications match what appears within the **Medication Administration Record (MAR)** for this time period. If they do match, you can click the **Administer** icon. If they do not match, you should select **Hold Medications**. When you are finished, click **Continue Working With Patient** to return to the patient care menu.

■ VITAL SIGNS

Vital signs are often considered the traditional signs of life and include body temperature, heart rate, respiratory rate, blood pressure, oxygen saturation of the blood, and the patient's experience of pain.

Inside Carmen Gonzales' room, click on the **Vital Signs** icon. This icon activates a pathway that allows you to measure the patient's vital signs. When you enter this pathway, you will see a short video in which the nurse informs the patient what is about to happen. Six vital signs options appear at the bottom of the screen. Each icon activates a video clip in which the respective vital sign is measured. Relevant vital signs data become available in these videos. For example, click on **Heart Rate**, and a video clip and animation of a radial pulse appear. You can measure the heart rate by counting the animated pulses during a prescribed time.

Try each of the different vital signs options to see what kinds of data are obtained. The vital signs data change over time to reflect the temporal changes you would find in a patient similar to Carmen Gonzales. You will see this most clearly if you "leave" the Tuesday time period you are currently within and "come back" on Thursday. However, you will also find changes throughout any given day (for example, differences between the 0700–1100 and 1100–1500 shifts).

Collect vital signs data for Carmen Gonzales and enter them into the following table. Note the time at which you collected these data.

Vital Signs	Findings/Time
Blood Pressure	
O_2 Saturation	
Heart Rate	
Respiratory Rate	
Temperature	
Pain Rating	

After you are done, click on the **3rd Floor** icon in the lower right portion of your screen. This will take you back into the hallway. Move along the hallway (or use the animated map in the upper right corner of your screen) to return to the Nurses' Station. Enter the station, and click on the computer that accesses the Electronic Patient Record (EPR). First you will see the Electronic Patient Record System entry screen. Type in **rn2b** for the password (remember, do *not* press the Return/Enter key). Then click **Access Records**, and you will see a new screen with patients listed. Click on **Carmen Gonzales** and then on **Access EPR**. Now you are in the EPR system. Click on **Vital Signs**, which will open the screen with vital signs data. Use the blue and orange arrows in the lower right-hand corner of the data table to move around within the database. Look at the data collected earlier for each of the vital signs you measured. Use these data to establish a baseline for each of the vital signs.

a. Are any of the data you collected significantly different from the baselines for those vital signs?	Circle One: Yes No
b. If "Yes," which data are different?	

■ PHYSICAL ASSESSMENT

After examining the EPR for vital signs, click the **Assessment** icon and review Carmen Gonzales' data in this area. Once you have reviewed the data and noted any areas of concern to you, close the EPR, enter Carmen Gonzales' room, and click on the **Physical** icon. This will activate the following three options for conducting a physical assessment of the patient:

- Head and Neck
- Chest/Upper Extremities
- Abdomen and Lower Extremities

Click on the **Head and Neck** icon. You will see the nurse conduct an assessment of the head and neck. At the end of the video, a series of icons appear in a frame to the right of the video screen. These icons list the different areas of the head and neck that were examined and the data obtained during the examination. The icons allow you to replay that section of the video in which the particular area was examined.

For example, if you click on **Oculomotor** (the finding is "Oculomotor function intact"), you will see a replay of the assessment of oculomotor function. Each of the icons activates only that portion of the head and neck assessment focused on the particular area described by the icon. The intention is to help you correlate each part of a physical assessment with the data obtained from that assessment—and to give you the opportunity to have the whole assessment of a region conducted beginning to end so that you can learn the process as well as its component parts. Click **Continue Working with Patient** and explore the Chest/Upper Extremities and the Abdomen and Lower Extremities options. For each area, browse through the icons that provide data on a particular area of the assessment. *(Note: The data for certain attributes found during physical assessments change for some patients as you follow them through the virtual week.)*

Focus on the examination of the abdomen and lower extremities by clicking on the option. Pay close attention to the leg wound. In the following table, record the data collected by the nurse during the examination.

Area of Examination	Findings
Abdomen	
Legs	

After you have completed the physical examination of the abdomen and lower extremities, click **Continue Working with Patient** to return to the patient care menu. From there, click on the **3rd Floor** icon and return to the Nurses' Station. Enter the data you collected in Carmen Gonzales' EPR. Compare the data that were already in the record with the data you just collected.

a. Are any of the data you collected significantly different from the baselines for those vital signs?	Circle One: Yes No
b. If "Yes," which data are different?	

■ HEALTH HISTORY

Conduct part of a health history of Carmen Gonzales. Return to her room and click on the **Health History** icon. Twelve health history areas become visible as icons below the video screen. For example, you can see Perception/Self-Concept, Activity, Sexuality/Reproduction, and so on. Note that this patient speaks Spanish and that the nurse has brought in a translator. All of the health history conversations with Carmen Gonzales are completed through translation. Clicking on any of the 12 health history icons reveals three question areas for that category. For example, if you click **Perception/Self-Concept**, a box appears to the right of the video screen with three question areas:

- Impact of Hospitalization
- Fear and Anxieties
- Perception of Abilities

Each of these three areas can be activated by clicking on their respective icons. When an icon is clicked, you will see a video in which your preceptor asks a question in the respective area and the patient answers through the translator.

Since there are 12 health history areas, with three areas of questioning for each, you have access to a total of 36 video clips that provide an opportunity to learn quite a bit about Carmen Gonzales. The questions and responses were chosen for reasons. In fact, conducting an actual health history would not unfold in such discrete and isolated moments; in the real world you would need to follow up some responses with additional questions. Other lessons in this workbook will encourage you to look at each of the health history areas and decide what additional questions need to be asked.

Unlike the vital signs and physical examination findings, the health history data do not change. The developers of *Virtual Clinical Excursions* realized that the number of videos (and the space required for storage) would become too large for the type of educational package we envisioned. We therefore decided to produce only one set of health history data-collecting opportunities. In truth, the health history would probably not change much over a week. Lessons in your workbook may have you collect health history data on the first day of care, or some of the health history queries may be assigned for Tuesday and the others for Thursday.

We recommend that you explore the health history of Carmen Gonzales by choosing some of the 12 categories and asking one or two of the three questions available for each area. When you are done exploring the health history options, leave the patient's room and go to one of the computers that allow you to access the EPR. Browse through the different data fields to see where you would enter data from the health history questions.

Remember: When you are ready to stop working with your *Virtual Clinical Excursions Patients' Disk*, click on the **Quit** icon found in the lower right-hand corner of any of the 3rd floor screens.

■ COLLECTING AND EVALUATING DATA

Each of the patient care activities generates a great deal of assessment data. Remember that after you collect data, you can go to the Nurses' Station or the mobile computer outside Room 302 and enter the data into the EPR. You also can review the data in the EPR, as well as review a patient's chart and MAR. You will get plenty of practice collecting and then evaluating data in the context of the patient's course during previous shifts.

Now, here's an important question for you:

> Did the previous sequence of exercises provide the most efficient way to assess Carmen Gonzales?

For example, you went to the patient's room to get vital signs, then back to the EPR to enter data and compare your finding with extant data. Then, you went back to the patient's room to do a physical examination, and again back to the EPR to enter and review data. If this back-and-forth process of data collection and recording seemed inefficient, remember the following:

- You want to plan all of your nursing activities to maximize efficiency while at the same time optimizing quality of patient care.
- You collect a tremendous amount of data when you work with a patient. Very few people can accurately remember all these data for more than a few minutes. Develop efficient assessment skills, and enter assessment data as soon as possible after collecting them.
- Assessment data are only the starting point for the nursing process.

Make a clear distinction between these first exercises and how you actually provide nursing care. These initial exercises were designed to involve you actively in the use of different software components. This workbook focuses on sensible practices for implementing the nursing process in ways that ensure the highest quality care of patients.

Most importantly, remember that a human being changes through time—and that these changes include both the physical and psychosocial facets of a person as a living organism. Think about this for a moment. Some patients may change physically in a very short time (a patient with emerging myocardial infarction) or more slowly (a patient with chronic illness). Patients' overall physical and psychosocial conditions may improve or deteriorate. They may have effective coping skills and familial support or feel they are alone and full of despair. In fact, each individual is a complex mix of physical and psychosocial elements, and at least some of these elements usually change through time.

Thus it is crucial *not* to think of the nursing process as a simple one-time, five-step procedure:

- Assessment
- Nursing Diagnosis
- Planning
- Implementation
- Evaluation

Rather, it is a creative and systematic approach to delivering nursing care. Furthermore, because all living organisms are constantly changing, we must apply the nursing process over and over. Each time we follow the nursing process for an individual patient, we refine our understanding of that patient's physical and psychosocial conditions based on collection and analyses of many different types of data. *Virtual Clinical Excursions* will help you develop both the creativity and the systematic approach needed to become a nurse who can deliver the highest quality care to all patients.

The following icons are used throughout the workbook to help you quickly identify particular activities and assignments:

 Indicates a reading assignment—tells you which textbook chapter(s) you should read before starting each lesson

 Indicates a writing activity

 Marks the beginning of an interactive CD-ROM activity—signals you to open or return to your *Virtual Clinical Excursions Patients' Disk*

 Indicates additional CD-ROM instructions

 Indicates questions and activities that require you to consult your textbook

LESSON **1**

Promoting Healthy Lifestyles

Reading Assignment: Promoting Healthy Lifestyles (Chapter 3)

Patients: Carmen Gonzales, Room 302
Ira Bradley, Room 309
Andrea Wang, Room 310

In this lesson you will examine various health promotion concepts and strategies and determine how they apply to three different patients. Before you begin, note that the chapter compares and contrasts health promotion, risk reduction, and disease prevention and discusses *Healthy People 2010* in the context of a national agenda for health promotion. The role of the nurse in health promotion is critically important to the health of individuals, families, and communities. For this reason, it is important to be able to recognize and act on opportunities to engage in health promotion activities with patients.

Review pp. 33 and 34 in your textbook. Then answer questions 1–3 below.

 Writing Activity

1. Briefly compare and contrast the textbook descriptions of health promotion, risk reduction, and disease prevention.

   a. Health promotion

   b. Risk reduction

c. Disease prevention

2. Briefly describe primary, secondary, and tertiary prevention.

a. Primary prevention

b. Secondary prevention

c. Tertiary prevention

3. To which of the above categories do you think most hospitalized patients belong? Explain your answer.

CD-ROM Activity

You will now review selected areas of the health history of three patients: Carmen Gonzales, Ira Bradley, and Andrea Wang. Open your *Virtual Clinical Excursions Patients' Disk*. First go to the Supervisor's Office and sign in to work with Carmen Gonzales on Tuesday at 0700. Next go to the patient's room (Room 302) to conduct a partial nursing history. Review the sections indicated below and answer question 4 on lifestyle patterns that impact health and wellness, such as usual dietary habits, food preferences and dislikes, usual exercise or activity levels, the patient's perception of her own health, and her ability to cope with stress.

- Click on **Health History**.
- Review each of the following four areas, one at a time: Nutrition-Metabolic, Activity, Health Perception, and Coping/Stress. Then review the subtopics within each category by clicking on each of them.
- As you listen, record your answers to question 4 on the next page.

4. Record data found in Carmen Gonzales' health history below.

Nutrition-Metabolic

Activity

Health Perception

Coping/Stress

→ When you are finished, click on the **3rd Floor** icon in the lower right-hand corner of the screen to leave the room. Return to the Supervisor's Office and sign in to work with Ira Bradley on Tuesday at 0700. Then go to his room (Room 309) to conduct a partial health history, just as you did with Carmen Gonzales.

- Click on **Health History**.
- Review each of the following four areas, one at a time: Nutrition-Metabolic, Activity, Health Perception, and Coping/Stress. Then review the subtopics within each category by clicking on each of them.
- As you listen, record your answers to question 5.

5. Record data found in Ira Bradley's health history below and on the next page.

Nutrition-Metabolic

Activity

Health Perception

Coping/Stress

→ Return to the Supervisor's Office. Sign in to work with Andrea Wang on Tuesday at 0700. Go to Room 310 to conduct a partial nursing history, just as you did with the two previous patients.

- Click on **Health History**.
- Review each of the following four areas, one at a time: Nutrition-Metabolic, Activity, Health Perception, and Coping/Stress. Then review the subtopics within each category by clicking on each of them.
- As you listen, record your answers to question 6 below.

6. Record data found in Andrea Wang's health history below.

Nutrition-Metabolic

Activity

Health Perception

Coping/Stress

Writing Activity

Recall that Chapter 3 discusses the issue of physical activity and rest and also emphasizes diet and nutrition. Use information from these textbook sections and findings from the previous patients' histories to answer the following questions.

7. Which of these patients has the least healthy baseline dietary pattern? Discuss the rationale for your answer and compare this patient's dietary pattern with those of the other two patients. *Hint:* Refer to the section entitled "Promoting a Healthy Diet" on pp. 45-47 of your textbook, as well as Figure 3-1, The USDA Food Guide Pyramid, and Table 3-5, Dietary Guidelines for Americans.

8. For each of these three patients, identify a current barrier to maintaining an optimal level of physical activity.

Carmen Gonzales

Ira Bradley

Andrea Wang

9. All three patients you have visited have serious stressors related to illness. Stressors can have a negative effect on mental health and interfere with rest and sleep. Identify a major stressor described by each patient during the nursing history.

Carmen Gonzales

Ira Bradley

Andrea Wang

We will now look more closely at the nutritional status of two patients.
- Return to the Supervisor's Office, and sign in to work with Carmen Gonzales on Tuesday at 1100. Go to the Nurses' Station and open her chart. Click on **History and Physical** and note her height and weight on p. 3 of that report. Record this data in question 10 below.
- Return to the Supervisor's Office again, and sign in to work with Ira Bradley on Tuesday at 1100. Find Ira Bradley's height and weight as you did for Ms. Gonzales and record it in question 10 below.

 10. Now estimate the body mass index (BMI) for Carmen Gonzales and Ira Bradley. *Hint:* Use the Body Mass Index chart on p. 44 of the textbook. Refer to the legend at the bottom of the chart to form a conclusion about the weight status of each patient (underweight, healthy weight, overweight, or obese). Record these answers below.

Patient	Height	Weight	BMI	Weight Status
Carmen Gonzales				
Ira Bradley				

 Knowledge of a healthy diet is needed as a basis for conducting dietary teaching. Review in your textbook Figure 3-1, The USDA Food Guide Pyramid, and Table 2-2, Dietary Guidelines for Americans. Match each of the following dietary guidelines with its corresponding food item. Note that more than one food item may apply to a dietary guideline.

Dietary Guideline	Food Item
11. _____ The daily diet should contain equal to or less than 30% of calories from this nutrient.	a. Vegetables
	b. Meat
12. _____ The daily diet should contain less than 10% of calories from this type of nutrient.	c. Fiber
13. _____ There should be three or more servings of this food item in the daily diet.	d. Saturated fat
	e. Salt
14. _____ There should be two or more servings of this food item in the daily diet.	f. Fruit
15. _____ There should be six or more servings of this food item in the daily diet.	g. Fat
	h. Milk
16. _____ The daily diet should include 20 to 30 grams of this item.	i. Grain products
17. _____ This type of item should be used in moderation in the daily diet.	j. Sugar
	k. Water
18. _____ Daily intake should include 5 to 8 glasses of this beverage.	

Chronic Illness

 Reading Assignment: Chronic Illness (Chapter 5)

Patient: Ira Bradley, Room 309

Chronic illness differs from acute illness in several ways. As a nurse, it is important to understand these differences to provide quality nursing care. In this lesson you will explore chronic illness as experienced by Ira Bradley and his family. Mr. Bradley has acquired immunodeficiency syndrome (AIDS), an incurable viral infection that ultimately leads to death.

Writing Activity

1. Compare and contrast the textbook definitions of acute illness and chronic illness. *Hint:* Refer to textbook p. 71.

2. What are two criteria used to define chronic illness on the National Health Survey?

    a.

    b.

3. What are four characteristics of chronic illness, according to the Commission on Chronic Illness?

    a.

    b.

    c.

    d.

CD-ROM Activity

Go to the Supervisor's Office and sign in to work with Ira Bradley on Tuesday at 0700. Next, go to the Nurses' Station and select his chart. Click on **History and Physical** and read the report. Then go to Ira Bradley's room to obtain a health history database. To do this, click on **Health History** and complete each section of the interview.

4. Record significant data for each of the health history areas below and on the next page.

Health History Area	Ira Bradley's Data
Perception/Self-Concept	
Activity	
Sexuality/Reproduction	
Culture	
Nutrition-Metabolic	
Sleep-Rest	

Health History Area	Ira Bradley's Data
Role/Relationship	
Health Perception	
Elimination	
Cognitive/Perceptual	
Coping/Stress	
Value/Belief	

5. The financial costs of managing chronic illness are often a heavy burden to families who have an ill family member. Besides private health insurance, what option(s) might Ira Bradley have for financial assistance with medical bills? *Hint:* See p. 74 of the textbook.

6. The textbook identifies four stages in the natural history of chronic disease. From what you have learned about Ira Bradley thus far, circle the stage that best describes his current situation. *Hint:* See textbook p. 76.

   Susceptibility   Presymptomatic disease   Clinical disease   Disability

7. There are many definitions of family. What type of family is Ira Bradley part of?

8. Family adaptability affects how successful a family is in managing changes brought about by a chronically ill family member. How adaptable are Ira Bradley and his wife, given the information you have gathered to this point? Briefly explain your answer.

9. How might Ira Bradley's wife benefit from having respite care for her husband?

Writing Activity

10. The textbook describes gender differences and how they relate to the caregiving role. Compare and contrast the information on p. 79 in your textbook about wives in the caregiving role with what you have learned about Ira Bradley's wife in this role.

11. Discuss the adequacy of available social supports that could decrease the feelings of burden and social isolation for Ira Bradley and his wife.

12. Below are five key assessment areas for the nurse as suggested by family stress theory. For each area identified, record the data for Ira Bradley and his wife based on what you have learned about them.

   a. What does Ira Bradley's illness mean to the family? Are there different meanings among the family members?

   b. What family characteristics serve as indicators of possible coping resources?

   c. What family characteristics suggest possible deficits in family coping?

   d. Has Ira Bradley's illness increased or decreased the family's cohesion? Briefly explain.

   e. Which religious beliefs and practices must be integrated into the plan of care?

 13. What is chronic grief? Offer an opinion about the risk for Ira Bradley and his family experiencing chronic grief. *Hint:* Refer to textbook p. 82 if needed.

14. What can be done to assist Ira Bradley and his family in dealing with chronic grief?

15. The phases of chronic illness, according to the chronic illness trajectory framework, are listed below. Circle the phase that best relates to Ira Bradley. Below the list of phases, briefly explain the rationale for your choice and identify a goal of management for the phase you chose. *Hint:* See Table 5-1 on p. 86 of the textbook.

Trajectory Phases:

Pretrajectory	Unstable	Comeback
Trajectory onset	Acute	Downward
Stable	Crisis	Dying

Rationale:

Goal of Management:

Loss, Grief, Dying, and End of Life Care

👓 **Reading Assignment:** Loss, Grief, Dying, and End of Life Care (Chapter 6)

Patients: Andrea Wang, Room 310
Ira Bradley, Room 309

In this lesson you will explore the meanings of loss and grief as they apply to two patients, Andrea Wang and Ira Bradley. Andrea Wang was paralyzed as a result of a diving accident. Ira Bradley has acquired immunodeficiency syndrome (AIDS), an incurable viral infection that ultimately leads to death. Both patients are experiencing significant but different losses and are in need of skillful assessment and care.

1. How is *loss* defined in the textbook?

2. Explain how loss can result in a crisis.

💿 **CD-ROM Activity**

Go to the Supervisor's Office and sign in to work with Andrea Wang on Tuesday at 0700. Go to the Nurses' Station and open her chart. Click on **History and Physical** and read the entire report. Next, click on **Nurses' Notes** and read all entries.

3. Is Andrea Wang experiencing a developmental or situational crisis? Explain.

Close Andrea Wang's chart and go to her room to conduct a complete health history. Review all of the sections to obtain a full database and holistic assessment of her experience of loss and grief. As you proceed, record the data in question 4 below and on the next page.

4. Record data from Andrea Wang's health history for each of the assessment areas.

Health History Section	Andrea Wang's Data
Perception/Self-Concept	
Activity	
Sexuality/Reproduction	
Culture	
Nutrition-Metabolic	
Sleep-Rest	
Role/Relationship	
Health Perception	
Elimination	
Cognitive/Perceptual	

Health History Section	Andrea Wang's Data

Coping/Stress

Value/Belief

5. A variety of factors influence the intensity and threat of a given loss. For each of the individual factors reproduced below from Box 6-1 of the textbook, place an X in the "Yes" column if this factor is likely to intensify her loss, in the "No" column if the factor is not likely to intensify it, or in the "Uncertain" column if you have insufficient data to draw a conclusion.

Factor	Yes	No	Uncertain
Age	_____	_____	_____
Personality	_____	_____	_____
Developmental level	_____	_____	_____
Past experience	_____	_____	_____
Role modeling	_____	_____	_____
Perception of intensity of loss	_____	_____	_____
Meaning of attachment	_____	_____	_____
Types of loss	_____	_____	_____
Replaceability	_____	_____	_____
Timing of experience	_____	_____	_____
Disruption from loss	_____	_____	_____
Threat to self and significant other(s)	_____	_____	_____
Coping skills	_____	_____	_____
Availability of support	_____	_____	_____

6. Discuss how a nurse's view of the professional nursing role as curative can increase occupational stress relating to loss.

7. How is grief related to loss?

8. In what stage of grief, as described by Kübler-Ross, is Andrea Wang? Briefly explain your answer.

9. List five general nursing interventions that may be helpful to Andrea Wang based on her identified stage of grief. *Hint:* Use the Guidelines for Safe Practice chart on p. 101 in your textbook to formulate an answer.

   a.

   b.

   c.

   d.

   e.

You will now explore loss and grief as experienced by another patient, Ira Bradley. Return to the Supervisor's Office and sign in to work with Ira Bradley on Tuesday at 1100. Go to the Nurses' Station and select his chart. Read the History and Physical and Nurses' Notes, as you did for Andrea Wang. Then answer questions 10, 11, and 12.

10. Is Ira Bradley experiencing a developmental or situational crisis? Explain.

11. Describe how loss can affect a family. *Hint:* Refer to textbook pp. 91–92 if needed.

12. Because of Ira Bradley's age, describe his expected concept of death and its potential impact. *Hint:* Refer to textbook p. 93 if needed.

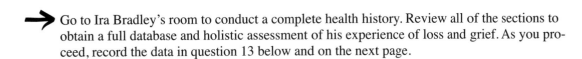 Go to Ira Bradley's room to conduct a complete health history. Review all of the sections to obtain a full database and holistic assessment of his experience of loss and grief. As you proceed, record the data in question 13 below and on the next page.

13. Record data from Ira Bradley's health history for each assessment area.

Health History Section	Ira Bradley's Data
Perception/Self-Concept	
Activity	
Sexuality/Reproduction	

Health History Section	Ira Bradley's Data
Culture	
Nutrition-Metabolic	
Sleep-Rest	
Role/Relationship	
Health Perception	
Elimination	
Cognitive/Perceptual	
Coping/Stress	
Value/Belief	

14. In which of Kübler-Ross's stages of grieving is Ira Bradley? Briefly explain your answer.

15. There are multiple dimensions of loss (listed below), and an individual may show specific manifestations of grief related to each of these dimensions. For each dimension listed, identify one or more manifestations that apply to Ira Bradley, based on your assessment. *Hint:* Refer to Box 6-2 on p. 94 for assistance if needed.

Physical

Cognitive

Psychologic

Social

Spiritual

16. Ira Bradley indicates he is of the Jewish faith. What is the typical meaning of death and dying to those in this cultural group? *Hint:* Refer to Table 6-3 on p. 98 if needed.

17. From what you have learned about Ira Bradley, identify a nursing diagnosis that relates to his and his family's loss.

18. Refer to the stage of grieving applicable to Ira Bradley that you identified in question 14. List at least six nursing interventions specific to his stage of grief that could be helpful to Ira Bradley. *Hint:* See textbook pp. 101–102 if needed.

    a.

    b.

    c.

d.

e.

f.

19. How might an advance directive or durable power of attorney be of use to Ira Bradley? *Hint:* Refer to p. 106 in the textbook if needed.

LESSON **4** _____

Emergency Care

_____

 Reading Assignment: Emergency Care (Chapter 7)

Patient: David Ruskin, Room 303

This lesson focuses on the emergency department (ED) as a health care delivery setting for David Ruskin, a patient admitted with possible closed head injury and fractured right humerus after being involved in a car-bicycle accident. From a review of textbook Chapter 7 and Mr. Ruskin's ED record, you will explore how care delivered in this setting helps patients to achieve health goals.

 Review in your textbook the section entitled "Scope of Practice for Emergency Nursing" on pp. 118–122. Then complete the following questions and matching exercise.

✎ **Writing Activity**

1. The textbook indicates that triage is a function in all emergency departments. Describe the origin and meaning of the word *triage*.

2. Briefly describe each of the following triage labels used to categorize patients in the ED according to acuity level.

Emergent

Urgent

Nonurgent

In times of disaster, a color-coded triage system may be used. Match each of the following descriptions of patient injuries with the corresponding triage color code.

Description of Patient Injuries	Triage Color Code
3. _____ Ambulatory with minor cuts and lacerations; in a dazed state	a. Black
	b. Red
4. _____ Burn injury on anterior chest and a closed fracture of the arm that has been immobilized	c. Yellow
5. _____ Dead	d. Green
6. _____ Severe abdominal injury and difficulty breathing	

7. Describe the uses and benefits of critical pathways in the emergency department.

8. There are legal and forensic considerations in emergency nursing practice. Give three examples of situations in which the nurse may be required by state and local laws to engage in mandatory reporting.

a.

b.

c.

CD-ROM Activity

You will now conduct a brief review of the medical record for David Ruskin, who was admitted via the emergency department after sustaining multiple trauma.

- Go to the Supervisor's Office and sign in to work with David Ruskin on Thursday at 1100. Next go to the Nurses' Station and find Mr. Ruskin's chart.
- Open the chart and click on **History and Physical**. Read the Emergency Department Report and the History and Physical to get a broad idea of the important findings.
- As you read the Emergency Department Report, think about the components of the primary and secondary surveys, as illustrated in Figure 7-1 of your textbook.
- When you have finished, review the report once again. This time, record the information you read on the Trauma Flow Sheet on the next two pages. *Note:* There will not be enough information to fill in every section of the flow sheet.

9. Fill in data from David Ruskin's Emergency Department Record on the primary and secondary survey flow sheet below and on the next page.

Red Rock Canyon Medical Center	
Emergency Medical Services **Trauma Flow Sheet**	**Patient Name Label**

Date: _____

~~**Arrival time:**~~ ___:___ Injury time ___:___ Transferred from: _____

Arrived by: Helicopter: _____ Squad: _____ ALS/BLS

Documentation received: ER Record   X-Rays   CT Scan

Mechanism: **MVA:** Driver/Passenger   Location in vehicle: _____ Carseat Y/N

Restraint: Type: _____ Vehicle damage: _____

Vehicle speed: High/Low   Rollover   Ejected   Head-on   T-Bone   Rear-end

Pedestrian struck/Fall: Speed of vehicle/Height of fall: _____

GSW/stab: Caliber/Size of weapon: _____ Distance: _____

Other: _____

Past Medical HX: Cardiac   Renal   Respiratory   HTN   Diabetic   Other: _____

Medications: _____

Allergies: _____ **Approx. wt:** _____ kg

Last menses: _____   **Last tetanus:** _____

HPI: _____
_____
_____

Family Notification: Notified/Enroute   Phone consent Y/N   Unable to notify   Present

Contact person: _____   Phone: _____

Prehospital Intervention

Airway: Oral/Nasal Combi Intubated

O₂: High flow Cannula None BVM

IV Access: GA_____ Total fluid _____

IV Access: GA_____ Total fluid _____

Immobilized: Y/N

CPR: Y/N Time begun:__:__

Procedure: _____

Procedure: _____

Response			
Service	**Time**	**PTA**	**Name**
Trauma res	__:__	__	_____
Trauma chief	__:__	__	_____
Neurosurgery	__:__	__	_____
Anesthesia	__:__	__	_____
Radiology	__:__	__	_____
E.R. Attending	__:__	__	_____
Surg. Attending	__:__	__	_____

Primary Survey

Airway: Patent Obstructed

Intervention: Oral/Nasal Airway size _____ MM

Intubated: Oral/Nasal size_____ MM Depth _____ CM

Procedure: Cric size _____ MM Depth _____ CM

Breathing: No Distress Distressed <10 >26 Assisted BVM/Vent

Expansion: Symmetrical/Asymmetrical Flail R/L Tracheal Deviation R/L

Intervention: O₂-high flow   Assisted — BVM

Chest tube R/L Size _____ FR   Amt out_____ CC

Chest tube R/L Size _____ FR   Amt out_____ CC

Circulation: Skin — Warm Dry Moist Cool Pink Pale Cyanotic

Cap refill — Brisk Delayed None

Pulses Present: All present Deficit_____

Obvious Bleeding site_____

Intervention: Bleeding control

IV Access: Cent/Periph site _____ GA _____ NS/LR by _____

IV Access: Cent/Periph site _____ GA _____ NS/LR by _____

Procedure: Thoracotomy   ACLS Protocol   ATLS Protocol

Other: _____

Disability: Awake   Responds to verbal   Responds to pain   Unresponsive

T R A U M A   F L O W   S H E E T

Secondary Survey   Time: ___:___

Date: _____

Neuro:
Mental status: A V P U   GCS: E__ V__ M__
Pupils: R __ L __ EOM: Intact Deficit _____
Drainage: Nasal Ears R/L Clear/Bloody None
Motor and sensory: Grossly intact Deficits _____
Other: _____

Respiratory:
Trachea: Midline Deviated R/L
Chest expansion: Symmetrical/Asymmetrical Flail R/L
Resp effort: Unlabored 12-18/min Distressed <10 >26 Absent
Breath sounds: R _____ L _____
Other: _____

Cardiovascular:
Skin: Warm/Dry Other_____
Cap refill: Normal Delayed
Pulses: All present Deficit _____
Heart sounds: S1, S2 Rub Murmur Other_____
Other: _____

GI/GU:
Abd: Soft/Nontender Flat Firm Rigid Distended Tender _____
Pelvis: Stable Unstable
Bowel sounds: Y/N Other_____
Rectal: Heme: +/− Tone: NL Flaccid
Blood at urinary meatus: Y/N
Other: _____
Skeletal: _____

Pupil Gauge
2	3	4	5	6	7	8	9

Pupil Gauge
Diameter by millimeter

Glasgow Coma Score
Eyes	Open spontaneously	4
	To verbal command	3
	To painful stimuli	2
	No response	1
Verbal	Oriented and converses	5
	Disoriented and converses	4
	Inappropriate words	3
	Incomprehensible sounds	2
	No response	1
Motor	Obeys command	6
	Localizes pain	5
	Flexion/Withdrawal	4
	Flexion/Abnormal	3
	Extension	2
	No response	1

Interventions
Time

__:__ Cardiac monitor
__:__ NIPB
__:__ Pulse oximeter
__:__ 12 LD EKG
__:__ Foley size __ Heme +/−
__:__ NG/OG size __ Heme +/−
__:__ ICP bolt
__:__ A-line- Rad R/L Fem R/L

__:__ DPL
__:__ Warming _____

Radiology
Time in Time out

Portable C-spine, Pelvis,
__:__ __:__ Chest
__:__ __:__ Plain films
__:__ __:__ CT _____
__:__ __:__ A-Gram _____
__:__ __:__ Repeat _____
__:__ __:__ Repeat _____

__:__ C:spine cleared by: _____
__:__ C-collar removed by: _____
__:__ Backboard removed by: _____

Pediatric Coma Scale
Eye Opening
Spontaneous	4
To verbal command or shout	3
To pain	2
No response	1

Best Verbal Response
> 5 years
Oriented and converses	5
Disoriented and converses	5
Inappropriate words	3
Incomprehensible sounds/garbled	2
No response	1

2-5 years
Appropriate words and phrases	5
Inappropriate words	4
Cries, screams	3
Moans, grunts	2
No response	1

0-23 months
Smiles, coos, cries appropriately	5
Cries	4
Inappropriate crying, screaming	3
Moans, grunts	2
No response	1

Best Motor Response
Obeys commands	6
Localizes pain	5
Withdraws (normal flexion)	4
Abnormal flexion (decorticate)	3
Extension (decerebrate)	2
No response	1

Musculoskeletal

A = Abrasion	H = Hematoma
B = Burn	L = Laceration
D = Deformity	M = Amputation
E = Ecchymosis	P = Penetrating
F = Foreign body	T = Tenderness
	Av = Avulsion

Rule of Nines

Burns

18 Front
18 Back
9 9
18 18

18
18 Front
18 Back
14 14
9 9

10. Review your descriptions of triage categories in question 2. To which of these categories did David Ruskin belong at the time of admission to the ED?

In the section entitled "Prevention of Trauma" on pp. 122–123 of your textbook, six types of accidents are outlined. For each of them, preventive measures are also discussed. Review this information and answer question 11 below.

11. For each of the following types of accidental injuries, list one or more preventive measures.

Type of Unintentional Injury	Preventive Measure(s)
Motor vehicle accidents	
Falls	
Burns	
Accidental poisonings	
Head injuries in pedal cyclists	
Scooter injuries	

12. Was David Ruskin using appropriate preventive measures at the time of his injury? Provide a brief rationale for your answer.

13. Emergency departments have specific designations to indicate their status for trauma care. Briefly define each of the three levels of trauma centers.

Level I

Level II

Level III

14. Based on what you know about David Ruskin, form an opinion as to what level of trauma center would have adequately met his needs for care. Briefly explain the rationale for your answer.

15. An accidental injury can be a time of crisis for the family as well as the patient. If you were the nurse in the emergency department, what interventions could you use to offer support to Mr. Ruskin's wife Lisa? *Hint:* Refer to p. 130 of your textbook for suggestions if needed.

LESSON **5**

Inflammation and Infection

 Reading Assignment: Inflammation and Infection (Chapter 11)

Patients: Carmen Gonzales, Room 302
Sally Begay, Room 304

In this lesson you will apply concepts related to inflammation and infection to the assessment and care of two patients. The first patient is Carmen Gonzales, admitted to the hospital with a left lower leg wound complicated by gangrene infection and osteomyelitis. The second is Sally Begay, who was admitted with a rule out diagnosis of Hantavirus that was subsequently changed to pneumonia. It may be helpful to have a medical dictionary and laboratory/diagnostic test handbook available for use during this lesson.

Writing Activity

1. Compare and contrast the terms *inflammation* and *infection*. *Hint:* Refer to p. 183 of the textbook.

2. Identify the specific and nonspecific defenses that the body uses to prevent and combat infection.

Specific

Nonspecific

 Match each of the following steps in the inflammatory response with the mediators of that response. *Hint:* Use Table 11-1 on p. 184 if needed.

Mediators	**Step in the Inflammatory Response**
3. _____ Activation of clotting mechanism	a. Injury
4. _____ Fibroblasts produce collagen fibers, tissue regeneration	b. Vascular dilation
5. _____ Chemotactic substances released by complement activation, clot formation, and injured cells	c. Fibrin clot formation
	d. Fluid exudation
6. _____ Physical, chemical, biologic, and immunologic stimuli	e. Leukocyte exudation
7. _____ Neutrophils and macrophages	f. Attack and engulfment of foreign materials
8. _____ Histamine, plasmin, serotonin, kinins, prostaglandins released or activated by injury	g. Healing
9. _____ Histamine, kinins, prostaglandins cause opening of venule-endothelial cell junction	

CD-ROM Activity

Go to the Supervisor's Office and sign in to work with Carmen Gonzales on Tuesday at 0700. Proceed to the Nurses' Station and open the patient's chart. Click on **History and Physical** and read the entire section, including the Emergency Department Record.

10. Identify three medical diagnoses that are listed upon admission in addition to the diagnoses of gangrene and osteomyelitis.

11. What are Ms. Gonzales' manifestations related to wound infection at the time of her presentation to the Emergency Department?

12. What are her vital signs on admission?

Temperature _____   Heart rate _____   Respiratory rate _____

Blood pressure _____

13. How does Carmen Gonzales' leg infection relate to her clinical findings? How can these findings be explained? Use the chart below to answer this question.

Clinical Findings	Explanation of the Findings
Fever	
Increased heart and respiratory rates	
Leg pain	

14. In the Emergency Department Record, the physician describes an area of necrosis on the medial side of Carmen Gonzales' left leg. What does the term *necrosis* mean? Refer to p. 186 in your textbook or a medical or nursing dictionary if needed.

15. What correlation could there be between Carmen Gonzales' other medical problems and the development of gangrene in this wound?

➤ Click on **Physicians' Orders** in Carmen Gonzales' chart. Read the orders for Sunday at 1830.

16. The physician ordered a CBC (complete blood count) and a wound culture. What are the rationales for these tests? *Hint:* Refer to pp. 204 and 206 in your textbook if needed.

➤ Close the chart. Access the computer under the bookshelf, and open the EPR for Carmen Gonzales. Click on **Hematology** and review the CBC and differential results on Sunday evening.

17. Record Carmen Gonzales' results from Sunday evening for each of the lab tests below.

Lab Test	Result	Lab Test	Result
Hgb		Neutrophil segs %	
Hct		Neutrophils bands %	
RBC		Lymphocytes %	
Platelets		Monocytes %	
WBC		Eosinophils %	
		Basophils %	

18. Identify any abnormal results recorded in question 17 and indicate whether each abnormal result is high or low. What is your interpretation of the CBC results? Are these results expected or unexpected? Refer to a laboratory or diagnostic test book for help if needed.

 Go to Ms. Gonzales' room to assess her leg wound. Click on **Physical Examination** and then on **Abdomen and Lower Extremities**. Examine the wound and take notes in the area below. Make note of any data related to circulation as well. When you have finished, click **Continue Working With Patient**.

Student Notes

 19. After noting the characteristics of Carmen Gonzales' wound, refer to Repair and Healing on p. 185 in your textbook. What stage of the healing process characterizes her leg wound? Provide a brief rationale for your answer.

Proper nutrition is essential for adequate healing of inflamed or infected tissue. While you are still in Carmen Gonzales' room, conduct a brief nutritional assessment by clicking on **Health History** and then on **Nutrition-Metabolic**. Use the space below to record any useful information obtained as you assess this health pattern. Use your own baseline knowledge about nutrition and information from Lesson 1 of this workbook as a point of reference.

Student Notes

 20. What food groups are missing from Carmen Gonzales' diet, adversely affecting the healing process? Explain your reasoning.

 Return to the Supervisor's Office and sign in to work with Sally Begay on Tuesday at 1100. Complete the following activities.

- Go to the Nurses' Station and open her chart. Click on **History and Physical** and read the entire report, noting the rule out diagnosis of Hantavirus.
- Because Hantavirus is a less common health problem not commonly discussed in nursing textbooks, you decide to investigate this illness on the hospital Intranet. Close the chart and move to the computer to the left of the bookshelf. Click on this computer to access the Red Rock Canyon Medical Center's Intranet.
- Review the information available after typing in this address for the CDC website: http://www.cdc.gov/ncidod/diseases/hanta/hps/noframes/othrsrce.htm

21. What is Hantavirus?

22. Using the diagram below, which outlines the links in the chain of infection, fill in each of the boxes to describe how Sally Begay could have contracted Hantavirus.

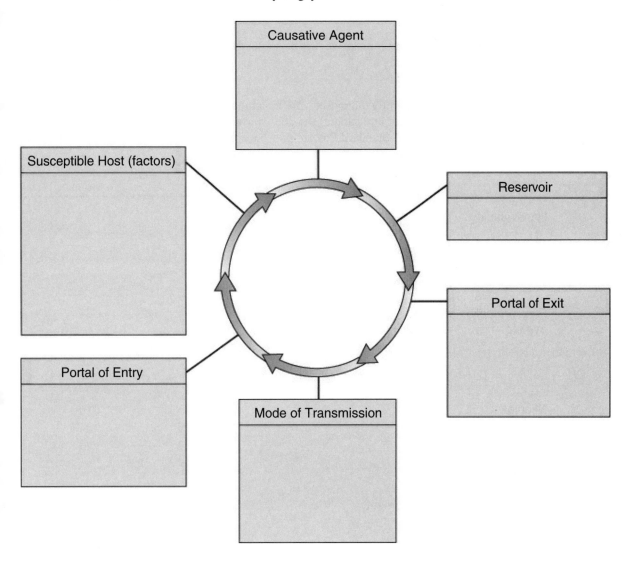

23. In addition to communicable infections, hospitalized patients are also at risk for nosocomial, or hospital-acquired, infections. Below and on the next page, place an X next to those factors that increase Sally Begay's risk for contracting a nosocomial infection. *Hint:* See p. 197 in the textbook if needed for descriptions of risk factors.

Predisposing Factor to Nosocomial Infection	Applies to Sally Begay
Age	_____
Impairment of normal immune defenses from underlying disease	_____
Impairment of normal immune defenses from therapy	_____
Use of antibiotics	_____
Use of invasive diagnostic and therapeutic procedures and devices	_____
Surgery	_____

Predisposing Factor to Nosocomial Infection	Applies to Sally Begay
Burns	_____
Lengthy hospitalization	_____
Severe underlying disease	_____

24. Sally Begay is subsequently diagnosed with pneumonia and has no need for transmission-based precautions. As for any patient, she does warrant use of Standard Precautions. Briefly describe the elements of Standard Precautions that are listed below. *Hint:* Use Table 11-8 on p. 202 if needed.

Element	Precautions
Handwashing	
Face protection (mask, eye protection, face shield)	
Needles	
Handling of reusable equipment	
Use of gloves	
Private room	
Handling of soiled linen	

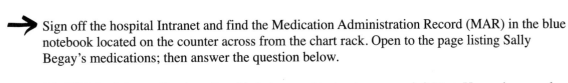 Sign off the hospital Intranet and find the Medication Administration Record (MAR) in the blue notebook located on the counter across from the chart rack. Open to the page listing Sally Begay's medications; then answer the question below.

25. Which of the medications listed is being used to treat pneumonia? *Hint:* Use a pharmacology or drug reference book if needed.

 26. The textbook lists five categories of general interventions for patients with infection. For each of the categories listed below, write in specific interventions that could be used when caring for Sally Begay. *Hint:* See pp. 209–210 of your textbook.

Category	Specific Interventions for Sally Begay
Promoting comfort	
Promoting normothermia	
Promoting adequate fluid volume	
Promoting rest	
Patient/family education	

LESSON 6

Pain

 Reading Assignment: Pain (Chapter 12)

Patients: Sally Begay, Room 304
David Ruskin, Room 303

In this lesson you will compare the pain experiences of two patients, Sally Begay and David Ruskin. Sally Begay is a 58-year-old Native American with a confirmed diagnosis of bacterial lung infection. David Ruskin is a 31-year-old patient who was injured after being hit by a car while bicycling. His injuries include a fractured humerus, chest contusion, and closed head injury.

Writing Activity

1. Read in the textbook the various definitions of pain. Briefly compare and contrast the definitions by Margo McCaffery and by the International Association for the Study of Pain.

 2. Identify at least five factors that can influence an individual's response to pain. *Hint:* Refer to Box 12-4 on p. 217 of your textbook if needed.

a.

b.

c.

d.

e.

65

3. Describe key differences between acute pain and chronic pain as they are discussed in your textbook. *Hint:* See Table 12-2 on p. 218 of your textbook.

🖥 CD-ROM Activity

Go to the Supervisor's Office and sign in to work with Sally Begay on Tuesday at 1100. Go to the Nurses' Station and open her chart. Click on **History and Physical** and read the report, making note below of any data related to pain.

Student Notes

 Click on **Nurses' Notes** and then **Expired MARS** and make note below of any data related to Sally Begay's pain or its treatment. Also find and list all the medications ordered for pain.

Student Notes

4. Review the section on pp. 209–210 in your textbook entitled "Specific Types of Pain." What type of pain is Sally Begay most likely experiencing? List the assessment data that you gathered to support your answer.

5. What documentation about pain is found in the History and Physical? Are these data supported by the documentation in the Nurses' Notes?

→ Now go to Sally Begay's room to do an assessment of your own. Click on **Vital Signs**.

6. Take a complete set of vital signs, making note of your findings here.

   Blood pressure _____   Temperature _____   Heart rate _____

   Respiratory rate _____   Oxygen saturation _____   Pain _____

7. When the nurse asks Ms. Begay to rate her pain, what type of assessment tool is she using? Refer to p. 226 in your textbook if needed.

8. Review the Assessment section in your textbook under Nursing Management, beginning on p. 226. List below the types of data that should be elicited during a pain assessment. Which of these pieces of data were collected for Sally Begay? Circle these. Which ones were omitted during this assessment? Underline these.

9. Write a nursing diagnosis for Sally Begay based on the data you have gathered thus far related to pain.

10. Identify outcome measures that could be used to evaluate the effectiveness of pain relief measures instituted for Sally Begay. Refer to the section entitled "Expected Patient Outcomes" on p. 229 in your textbook if you need help.

→ Go back to the Nurses' Station and open the MAR in the blue notebook on the counter. Review the current order for pain management for Sally Begay.

11. How many times has Sally Begay used medication for pain on this shift?

12. How many times has she used medication for pain since admission? Refer back to the notes you took earlier when reviewing the expired MARS if needed.

13. Of the three primary categories of analgesics discussed in the Pharmacological Approaches section of your textbook, which type of analgesic is ordered for Sally Begay?

14. What other types of medications belong to this same category?

15. Are you concerned about adverse effects from this analgesic medication? Explain your rationale.

16. What interventions other than analgesic medication are more likely to relieve Sally Begay's pain? Why? *Hint:* Review the section on medical management of pneumonia in Chapter 62 of your textbook if you are not familiar with this disorder.

→ Return to the Supervisor's Office and sign in to work with David Ruskin on Thursday at 1100. Go to the Nurses' Station and open his chart. Click on **History and Physical** and read the report, making note below of any data related to pain and how Mr. Ruskin perceives it.

Student Notes

_____

→ Next, click on **Nurses' Notes** and then on **Expired MARS** and make note of any data related to pain or its treatment. In addition, list all the medications that have been ordered for Mr. Ruskin's pain.

Student Notes

_____

➜ Now go to David Ruskin's room to do an assessment of your own. Click on **Vital Signs**.

17. Take a complete set of vital signs, making note of your findings here.

   Blood pressure _____ Temperature _____ Heart rate _____

   Respiratory rate _____ Oxygen saturation _____ Pain _____

18. When the nurse asks Mr. Ruskin to rate his pain, what type of assessment tool is she using?

19. Review the Assessment section in your textbook under Nursing Management, beginning on p. 226. List below the types of data that should be elicited during a pain assessment. Which of these pieces of data were collected on David Ruskin? Circle these. Which ones were omitted during this assessment? Underline these.

20. Write a nursing diagnosis for David Ruskin based on the data you have gathered thus far related to pain.

21. Identify outcome measures that could be used to evaluate the effectiveness of pain relief measures instituted for Mr. Ruskin. Refer to the section entitled "Expected Patient Outcomes" on p. 229 in your textbook if you need help.

→ Go back to the Nurses' Station and open David Ruskin's MAR in the blue notebook on the counter. Review the current order for pain management.

22. How many times has David Ruskin used medication for pain on this shift?

23. What pain medications are ordered for Mr. Ruskin, and what types of medications are they?

→ Now access Mr. Ruskin's EPR. Click on **Vital Signs** and locate data regarding his pain.

24. In the table below, record the rating, source, and characteristics of Mr. Ruskin's pain at the identified times.

	Sunday 2400	Tuesday 1600	Wednesday 2400
Pain rating			
Pain source			
Pain characteristics			

25. Based on an analysis of the data in the table above, how successful have the pain management interventions for Mr. Ruskin been to this point? Provide a rationale for your answer.

26. What three adverse effects of medication therapy could you anticipate for Mr. Ruskin, and what measures will you take to counteract them?

Fluid Imbalance

 Reading Assignment: Fluid, Electrolyte, and Acid-Base Imbalance (Chapter 13, pp. 236–249)

Patients: Ira Bradley, Room 309
        Carmen Gonzales, Room 302

In this lesson you will explore concepts and principles related to fluid balance and imbalance. You will apply this information to the care of a patient with fluid volume deficit (Ira Bradley) and one with fluid volume excess (Carmen Gonzales). Be sure to have a laboratory and diagnostic test reference book available as you complete this lesson.

Writing Activity

Review pages 236–244 in your textbook that discuss physiology of fluid and electrolyte balance and movement of fluids between body compartments. Then answer questions 1 through 11.

1. Identify the two fluid compartments in the body and describe their composition. *Hint:* Refer to p. 237 in your textbook.

2. Discuss the functions of body water.

Match each of the following terms related to fluid volume regulation with its corresponding definition.

Term	Definition
3. _____ Hydrostatic pressure	a. Passive transport of a solute across a membrane
4. _____ Colloidal osmotic pressure	b. The process used by the glomerular membrane of the kidney
5. _____ Filtration	
6. _____ Albumin	c. Movement of water from an area of higher water concentration to an area of lower water concentration
7. _____ Diffusion	
8. _____ Osmolarity	d. Pressure exerted against the wall of a blood vessel by the blood within it; also the pressure that exists within Bowman's capsule
9. _____ Aldosterone	
10. _____ Osmosis	e. The concentration of particles in 1000 mL of water
11. _____ Antidiuretic hormone	f. A hormone produced by the hypothalamus and released by the posterior pituitary gland to regulate body water

g. A common protein in the plasma that is responsible for pulling or absorbing fluid from the interstitial spaces

h. A hormone produced by the adrenal cortex that affects the kidneys' resorption of sodium and water in the renal tubules.

i. Pulls fluid back into the blood vessel from the interstitial space

CD-ROM Activity

Go to the Supervisor's Office and sign in to work with Ira Bradley on Tuesday at 0700. Next go to the Nurses' Station and open his chart. Click on **History and Physical** and read the Emergency Department Report and History and Physical. As you read, consider questions 12 and 13 and look for data that indicate possible fluid imbalance.

12. Below and on the next page, document any data you found in your chart review that could indicate possible fluid imbalance.

Emergency Department Report

History and Physical

13. Ira Bradley is diagnosed as being dehydrated. What precipitating factors does Mr. Bradley have for this condition?

➡ Now click on **Nurses' Notes** and read the note written by T. Landers on Sunday at 2335.

14. What subjective and objective date are found that relate to Mr. Bradley's fluid status?

➡ Click on **Physicians' Orders** and read the orders written on Sunday at 2255 hours.

15. List below any lab tests ordered to obtain further information about Ira Bradley's dehydration status. Also list any physician orders specifically written to treat and monitor the dehydration. Give a brief rationale for each. *Hint:* Use a laboratory and diagnostic test reference book as a guide if needed.

Laboratory Tests

Physician Orders

16. The textbook identifies three etiologies for fluid deficit on pp. 244 and 245. For each of the possible etiologies below, place an X in the appropriate column to indicate whether it does or does not apply to Mr. Bradley. Briefly explain each of your decisions.

Etiology	Applies	Does Not Apply	Rationale
Decreased fluid intake			
Fluid losses			
Sequestration of body fluids			

17. Listed below are the clinical manifestations of extracellular fluid depletion identified on p. 246 of the textbook. Based on the data you have obtained so far, place an X in the appropriate column to indicate whether or not Mr. Bradley exhibits each of these manifestations.

Clinical Manifestation	Exhibited by Mr. Bradley	Not exhibited by Mr. Bradley	Unable to Determine
Poor skin turgor			
Dry oral mucous membranes			
Postural hypotension			
Low blood pressure			
Tachycardia			
Increased respiration			
Decreased vein filling			
Weight loss			
Low urine output			
Increased urine specific gravity			

18. List four interventions that can be included in Mr. Bradley's care as part of collaborative management of fluid volume depletion. *Hint:* Refer to textbook pp. 246 and 247.

a.

b.

c.

d.

Return to the Supervisor's Office and sign in to work with Carmen Gonzales on Thursday at 0700. Go to the Nurses' Station and open her chart. Click on **Physicians' Notes** and read the entry for Tuesday at 1505. Note that the physician indicates congestive heart failure, a condition that relates to fluid volume excess. In question 19, record any data from the note pertaining to fluid volume status. Next, click on **Nurses' Notes** for Tuesday at 1530 and record data from that note pertaining to fluid status in question 19.

19. What data recorded in these sections of Ms. Gonzales' chart pertain to fluid volume status?

Physicians' Notes (Tuesday 1505)

Nurses' Notes (Tuesday 1530)

20. What other data indicative of fluid volume excess were not recorded in these parts of the chart? *Hint:* See pp. 247 and 248 in the textbook as needed.

➜ Close the chart and access Carmen Gonzales' EPR. Click on **I&O** and review the findings from the time of her surgery (Sunday at 2400) until Tuesday at 1200.

21. Add the numbers in the net column from Sunday at 2400 to Tuesday at 1200. How much fluid has Ms. Gonzales retained during this period of time? How does that relate to her clinical manifestations?

22. What other measurement of fluid volume status was conspicuously missing from the I&O section of the EPR for the entire duration of Ms. Gonzales' hospitalization?

23. Below, write specific suggestions for how to implement each of the listed interventions to treat fluid volume excess and assist Ms. Gonzales to recuperate from this episode. *Hint:* See p. 248 in the textbook for suggestions.

Intervention   **Suggestions on How to Implement**

Mobilize fluid

Reduce sodium intake

Reduce fluid intake

LESSON 8

Electrolyte Imbalance

Reading Assignment: Fluid, Electrolyte, and Acid-Base Imbalance (Chapter 13, pp. 236–244 and 249–269)

Patient: Ira Bradley, Room 309

In this lesson you will continue to work with Ira Bradley, who was admitted for dehydration, AIDS, *Pneumocystis carinii* pneumonia, and candidiasis. This time we will be exploring his electrolyte balance. As with the previous lesson, it may be helpful to have a laboratory and diagnostic test reference book available for use as you complete this lesson.

 Before you begin this lesson, review the introductory information about electrolytes on p. 237 in your textbook.

 Writing Activity

1. List nine electrolytes and identify each as a cation or an anion by placing an X in the appropriate column.

Electrolyte	Cation	Anion
a.		
b.		
c.		
d.		
e.		
f.		
g.		
h.		
i.		

2. Based on your reading, record the normal range in values for each of the serum (plasma) electrolytes listed below. Then indicate whether these electrolytes are found in greater quantities in the intracellular or extracellular fluid compartment. *Hint:* Use Table 13-1 on p. 237 in your textbook and a laboratory reference book for help.

Electrolyte	Normal Serum Range	Primary Compartment (Intracellular or Extracellular)
Sodium		
Potassium		
Chloride		
Calcium		
Ionized calcium		
Phosphorus (as phosphate)		
Magnesium		

 CD-ROM Activity

Go to the Supervisor's Office and sign in to work with Ira Bradley for the Tuesday 0700 shift. Proceed to the Nurses' Station, open his EPR, and click on **Chemistry**.

3. Find the laboratory test results for the Chem 7 that was done on Sunday at 2400. Record your findings below. Then indicate whether each value is low (L), high (H), or in the normal (N) range. Finally, indicate the significance of each result, if any (i.e., what might be causing the alteration). *Hint:* Refer to your answers in question 2 above, a laboratory reference book, and the Etiology paragraph for each electrolyte in the textbook.

Lab Test	Value	L, H, N	Significance of Result (if any)
Na^+			
K^+			
Cl^-			
CO_2			
BUN			
Creatinine			

Refer to pp. 251–252 in your textbook on hypernatremia to answer the following questions.

4. Identify and briefly describe two etiologies of hypernatremia. Which of these applies to Mr. Bradley, and why?

5. Summarize the following elements of the collaborative management of hypernatremia.

Preventive measures

Clinical manifestations to monitor

Fluid replacement

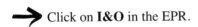 Click on **I&O** in the EPR.

6. By what route(s) was Ira Bradley's fluid replacement administered? Why was this appropriate?

7. How do you expect Mr. Bradley's serum sodium level to change as a result of the treatment you identified in question 6?

8. What would you measure to determine the effectiveness of the treatment you identified in question 6?

9. Return to question 3 in this lesson to find Mr. Bradley's serum potassium level. After reviewing the major etiologies for this electrolyte imbalance in your textbook, form a conclusion about which of them applies to Mr. Bradley. Provide a rationale for your answer.

10. Below, summarize the collaborative management of hyperkalemia.

Identification of those at risk

Clinical manifestations to monitor

Therapy for mild hyperkalemia

Therapy for severe hyperkalemia

11. Mr. Bradley can take clear liquids by mouth, and he has an order to advance diet as tolerated. Which beverages should Mr. Bradley avoid at this time because of potassium content? Use Table 13-9, Foods High in Potassium, on p. 254 in the textbook if needed.

→ It is now Friday and you are still interested in Ira Bradley's electrolyte status (and also with his fluid status, since they are interrelated); you wish to review how his care may have changed since Tuesday. Go to the Supervisor's Office and select Mr. Bradley as your patient on Friday at 1100. Remember, you will not be able to work with him during this time, but you will be able to review his progress. Go to the Nurses' Station and open his chart. Click on **Physicians' Orders**, **Physicians' Notes**, and **Nurses' Notes** and search for any documentation on Tuesday, Wednesday, or Thursday regarding his condition, change in status, or change in orders that particularly relate to his fluid and electrolyte imbalance.

12. Record below what you found in your chart review regarding Mr. Bradley's fluid and electrolyte status.

Source of data	Tuesday	Wednesday	Thursday
Physicians' Notes			
Physicians' Orders			
Nurses' Notes			

→ Close Mr. Bradley's chart and move to the computer under the bookshelf. Access the EPR and review Mr. Bradley's electrolytes and urine specific gravity over the entire week. (Click on **Chemistry** and **Urinalysis** to find these results).

13. Record your findings below and provide a rationale for any changes in the data. *Note:* You will also need to incorporate concepts from Lesson 7, Fluid Imbalance, to analyze this data appropriately.

Test	Sunday	Tuesday	Thursday	Rationale for Changes
Na^+				
K^+				
Cl^-				
CO_2				
BUN				
Creatinine				
Urine specific gravity				

Shock

 Reading Assignment: Shock (Chapter 14)

Patients: Carmen Gonzales, Room 302
Andrea Wang, Room 310

 In this lesson you will explore the condition of shock and the effects it may have on the health of two patients, Carmen Gonzales and Andrea Wang. Before beginning this lesson, review the pathophysiology of heart failure in Chapter 24 and spinal cord injury in Chapter 44 in your textbook.

Writing Activity

1. What is the definition of *shock* as presented in your textbook?

Below and on the following page, match each of the terms related to hemodynamic status with its corresponding definition.

Definition	**Term**
2. _____ The ventricular wall tension or stress during systolic ejection	a. Heart rate
	b. Cardiac output
3. _____ Resistance to blood flow created by the pulmonary arteries and arterioles, against which the right ventricle must pump	c. Preload
	d. Afterload
	e. Contractility
	f. Cardiac index
4. _____ Influenced by autonomic nervous system, increasing with sympathetic stimulation and decreasing with parasympathetic stimulation	g. Systemic vascular resistance
	h. Pulmonary vascular resistance
5. _____ The heart's contractile force or inotropy	i. Central venous pressure
6. _____ Pressure created by volume in the right side of the heart	j. Stroke volume

7. _____ The amount of blood the heart pumps per minute

8. _____ Cardiac output divided by the body surface area (to adjust for differences in body size)

9. _____ Amount of blood ejected by the ventricle with each heartbeat

10. _____ Resistance to blood flow created by the systemic vasculature against which the left ventricle must pump

11. _____ The amount of stretch in the ventricle at the end of diastole

12. Briefly describe the following three classifications of shock.

Hypovolemic

Cardiogenic

Distributive

13. What are the three types of distributive shock? Write a brief description of each.

 CD-ROM Activity

Sign in to work with Carmen Gonzales on Thursday at 1100 hours. Go to the Nurses' Station and open her chart. Click on **History and Physical** and review the entire report. As you read, consider question 14 below.

14. Which type of shock is Carmen Gonzales most at risk for developing? Explain your answer.

→ Close the chart and access the EPR for Carmen Gonzales. Click on **I&O** and scroll across the intake and output records for the week.

15. Did her fluid balance record from Sunday through Tuesday increase or decrease her risk of developing shock? Why?

→ Next, click on **Vital Signs** and review Carmen Gonzales' readings from Sunday through Tuesday.

16. To what extent do the vital signs exhibited by Carmen Gonzales fit the typical picture of a patient in shock? In what direction would the various vital sign measurements change if shock were present and progressing? *Hint:* Use Table 14-5 and the Pathophysiology of Shock section in Chapter 14 of your textbook for help.

17. How would a patient's urine output change if shock were present? Why?

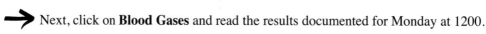 Next, click on **Blood Gases** and read the results documented for Monday at 1200.

18. What changes would you expect to see in the blood gas results if Carmen Gonzales were developing shock? *Hint:* Refer again to Table 14-5 in your textbook for help if needed.

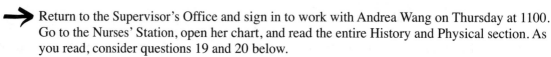 Return to the Supervisor's Office and sign in to work with Andrea Wang on Thursday at 1100. Go to the Nurses' Station, open her chart, and read the entire History and Physical section. As you read, consider questions 19 and 20 below.

19. Which type of shock is Andrea Wang most at risk for developing? Explain.

20. Note the vital signs documented in Andrea Wang's chart. Which of these results is consistent with the changes you would expect in a patient with shock, and which ones are not? Explain.

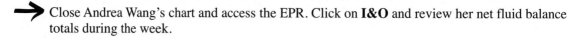 Close Andrea Wang's chart and access the EPR. Click on **I&O** and review her net fluid balance totals during the week.

21. Does Andrea Wang have a positive or negative net fluid balance as the week progresses? How does that affect the likelihood that she will develop shock? Explain your answer.

22. Central venous pressure (CVP) measurement is often the first invasive assessment made in the presence of shock. Using what you have learned so far about Carmen Gonzales and Andrea Wang and their risk factors for shock, discuss whether the CVP reading for each of them would rise or fall if shock were present. Explain.

23. The textbook outlines several treatments for shock; these are listed below. Under the column head for Carmen Gonzales, place an X next to each treatment that would be potentially useful for her. Now do the same for Andrea Wang in the third column. As you choose treatment options, keep in mind the etiology of the type of shock for which each of these women is at risk.

Treatment Used in Management of Shock	Useful for Carmen Gonzales?	Useful for Andrea Wang?
Oxygen therapy		
Drugs to improve cardiac output		
Intra-aortic balloon pump		
Ventricular assist device		
Pneumatic antishock garment (PASG)		
Surgical/invasive interventions		
Positioning supine with legs elevated		
Fluid resuscitation		
Blood administration		

24. Briefly summarize and discuss ways in which the overall treatment of shock is similar and different for Carmen Gonzales and Andrea Wang.

Similarities

Differences

 25. Identify four outcomes that would indicate effective collaborative management of shock that could be used for both Carmen Gonzales and Andrea Wang. *Hint:* Refer to p. 300 in your textbook.

LESSON 10

Preoperative Care

 Reading Assignment: Preoperative Nursing (Chapter 16)

Patient: David Ruskin, Room 303

In this lesson you will explore the preoperative experience of David Ruskin, who was injured when he was struck by a motor vehicle while riding a bicycle. He sustained a fractured right humerus and a closed head injury as a result of this trauma. He went to surgery for repair of the fracture to his arm.

In the left column below is a list of common suffixes related to surgical procedures. Match each suffix with its definition. *Hint:* Refer to Box 16-1 on p. 362 of the textbook if needed.

Suffix	**Definition**
1. _____ –ectomy	a. cutting into
2. _____ –rrhaphy	b. removal of an organ or gland
3. _____ –ostomy	c. providing an opening (stoma)
4. _____ –otomy	d. looking into
5. _____ –plasty	e. repairing
6. _____ –scopy	f. formation or plastic repair

7. What is the difference between a minimally invasive surgical procedure and an open surgical procedure?

8. What are the differences between a simple surgical procedure and a radical surgical procedure?

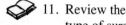 **CD-ROM Activity**

Go to the Supervisor's Office and sign in to work with David Ruskin at 0700 on Tuesday. Go to the Nurses' Station and open his chart. Click on **History and Physical** and read the Emergency Department Report.

9. What time did David Ruskin arrive in the emergency department?

10. What time did he go to surgery?

11. Review the paragraph on the purpose of surgical procedures on p. 363 in the textbook. What type of surgery did David Ruskin have, based on the purpose of his surgery?

12. Using the timing of surgery as a way of categorizing surgical procedures, was David Ruskin's surgery emergent, urgent, or elective? Explain.

13. Briefly describe the term *informed consent*. Give a brief explanation of why David Ruskin's wife Lisa signed the operative permit instead of Mr. Ruskin. *Hint:* Refer to the Informed Consent section on pp. 364–365 in your textbook if needed.

14. Important areas of data collection for the health history during the preoperative period are listed below. Using the Emergency Department Report and the History and Physical as your source, record the data collected from David Ruskin for each area. If an area was not completed, write "No data" in that section.

Areas of Data Collection	David Ruskin's Data
Allergies	
Medications and substance use	
Herbal and nutritional supplements	
Cultural and religious background	
Psychosocial status (support network)	
Functional assessment	
Level of anxiety	
Medical history	
Surgical and anesthetic history	
Perception of surgical procedure	
Perception of pain	

15. Why would it be important to gather further data about David Ruskin's reported allergy? What action should the nurse take after gathering this information?

16. Based on the data you have gathered thus far pertaining to David Ruskin, what is his physical classification according to the American Society of Anesthesiologists? *Hint:* Refer to Table 16-4 on p. 372 in the textbook. Briefly explain your answer.

17. In addition to data obtained from the health history, a physical examination provides necessary and important data for the preoperative assessment. For each of the physical exam areas listed below and on the next page, identify the key items to assess according to your textbook (pp. 376 and 378) in the middle column. In the last column, document the results from the Emergency Department assessments made on David Ruskin.

Physical Exam Area	Key Specific Assessments from Textbook	Assessments Made on David Ruskin
Cardiovascular		
Respiratory		
Renal		
Neurologic		

Physical Exam Area	Key Specific Assessments from Textbook	Assessments Made on David Ruskin
Musculoskeletal		
Integumentary		
Hydration		
Nutritional status		

18. If you were the nurse in the Emergency Department assigned to Mr. Ruskin, what preoperative teaching would you have provided? How would his level of consciousness have affected your teaching? *Hint:* Refer to the discussion on preoperative teaching on pp. 380–385 and Box 16-6 in the textbook if needed.

→ Click on **Physicians' Orders** in David Ruskin's chart. Read the list of orders written.

19. Preoperative medications are often given to patients before surgery, as outlined in Table 16-8 on pp. 385–386 of the textbook. Which of these medications did David Ruskin receive? Briefly summarize the action of the medication and any associated nursing implications.

20. What other medication did Mr. Ruskin receive that is not on this list? Give your opinion about why this medication was necessary.

→ Next click on **Surgeon's Notes** in the chart. Review the surgical note written for David Ruskin.

21. What time was David Ruskin brought into the operating room?

22. What time did his surgery actually begin?

23. What surgical procedure was performed?

24. How was the patient's fracture repaired?

25. What time did the surgical procedure end?

Postoperative Care

 Reading Assignment: Postoperative Nursing (Chapter 18)

Patient: David Ruskin, Room 303

In this lesson you will explore the postoperative experience of David Ruskin, who underwent surgery after being struck by a motor vehicle while riding a bicycle. Recall that he experienced a fractured right humerus and a closed head injury as a result of this trauma. Before beginning this lesson, be sure to complete Lesson 10, Preoperative Care, to become familiar with Mr. Ruskin's case.

Writing Activity

1. Briefly describe each of the following phases of care as identified by the American Society of PeriAnesthesia Nurses (ASPAN).

Preanesthesia phase

Postanesthesia phase I

Postanesthesia phase II

 2. When a patient is admitted to PACU, close and constant observation and assessment are essential for the recovery of the patient from anesthesia. What are the immediate nursing assessments upon admission to the PACU? *Hint:* Refer to Box 18-2 on p. 429 if needed.

CD-ROM Activity

Go to the Supervisor's Office and sign in to work with David Ruskin at 0700 on Tuesday. Go to the Nurses' Station and open his chart. Click on **Surgeon's Notes** and read the surgical report. According to the report, David Ruskin was transferred to the postanesthesia care unit (PACU) on Sunday at 1855.

3. The figure below illustrates PACU assessment using a body systems approach. In each of the boxes, fill in the assessments that should be made for David Ruskin while he is in PACU. *Hint:* See p. 430 of the textbook if needed.

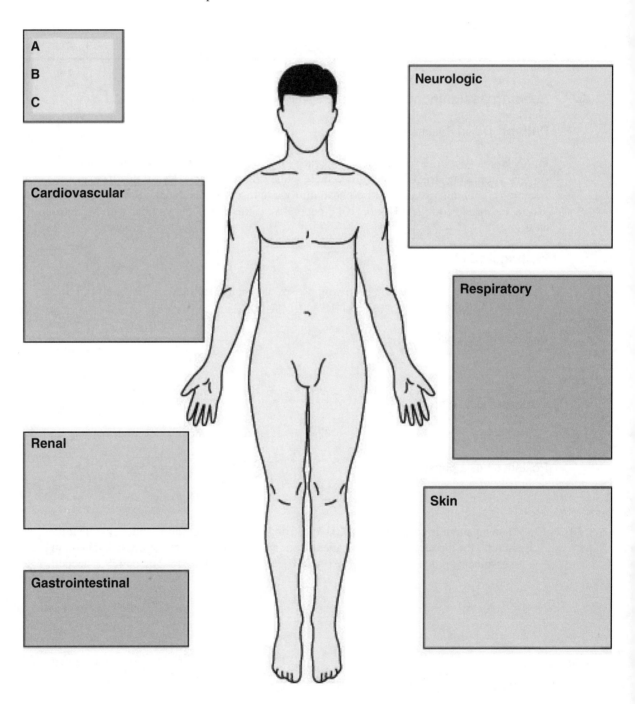

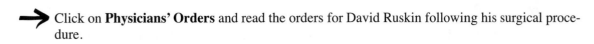 Click on **Physicians' Orders** and read the orders for David Ruskin following his surgical procedure.

    4. Pain is an important assessment in PACU as the patient recovers from anesthesia. What medication order was written for David Ruskin to treat his postoperative pain? Why is it ordered by the specified route?

    5. One major complication that occurs in the PACU is airway obstruction that could lead to hypoventilation. What clinical manifestations of airway obstruction would the PACU nurse assess for?

    6. If Mr. Ruskin developed any of the signs of airway obstruction noted in your answer to question 5, what initial actions should be taken? What interventions would need to be done if initial actions were unsuccessful?

7. Cardiac complications that could occur in PACU include hypotension, hypertension, and cardiac dysrhythmias. Define each of these complications. *Hint:* Refer to pp. 432–433 in the textbook if needed.

Hypotension

Hypertension

Cardiac dysrhythmias

➡ Click on **History and Physical** and note David Ruskin's baseline vital signs; then answer question 8 below. Record the vital signs below for quick reference as you proceed in the lesson.

Student Notes

_____

8. Refer to the definitions you wrote in question 7. What change in David Ruskin's systolic blood pressure would cause him to be hypotensive? What change would make him hypertensive? Calculate your answers below.

Hypotensive

Hypertensive

9. Hypothermia is a common disruption of thermoregulation during the surgical experience. List five adverse effects of hypothermia. *Hint:* See p. 433 of the textbook if needed.

   a.

   b.

   c.

   d.

   e.

→ Close the chart and open David Ruskin's EPR, located on the computer underneath the bookshelf. Click on **Vital Signs** and review the data recorded for Sunday at 2000.

10. What was David Ruskin's temperature upon admission to the surgical unit following discharge from PACU? Would this reading be considered hypothermic?

11. What was David Ruskin's blood pressure upon admission to the nursing unit following discharge from PACU? Would this reading be considered either hypotensive or hypertensive?

→ Click on **I&O** in the EPR to review David Ruskin's fluid volume status following transfer from PACU to the nursing unit. Review his oral and IV intake, as well as his net intake and output on Sunday at 2000.

12. Fluid volume replacement is essential postoperatively to replace fluid lost during surgery from blood loss and insensible losses via the lungs and skin. According to the data recorded for Sunday at 2000, what was David Ruskin's fluid intake during surgery and while he was in PACU? Record your answers below.

IV fluids:

IV antibiotics:

IV drips:

Total IV intake:

13. Find the fluid totals documented in the EPR on Sunday at 2000 as "In" and "Out." Which was greater, intake or output? By how much? Is this expected? Explain.

14. What are the possible consequences for Mr. Ruskin if this trend in fluid balance continues?

15. Using the Aldrete I scale, what criteria must be met before a patient can be discharged from PACU and transferred to the nursing unit? What is the total score needed for discharge from the PACU? *Hint:* See p. 434 and Table 18-1 on p. 438 in the textbook if needed.

Close the EPR and go to David Ruskin's room. Click on **Physical** and complete a full physical assessment on him, including Head and Neck, Chest/Upper Extremities, and Abdomen and Lower Extremities. Complete question 16 below as you proceed.

16. Listed below and on the next page are key postoperative assessments discussed in your textbook. Next to each area, record the data from David Ruskin's physical examination.

Area of Assessment	David Ruskin's Findings
Respiratory	
Cardiovascular	

Area of Assessment	David Ruskin's Findings
Gastrointestinal	
Urinary	
Wound status	
Pain	

17. Based on the specific data you obtained in question 16, identify and briefly explain two areas of continued priority assessment and care during David Ruskin's early postoperative period.

18. The textbook outlines postoperative care using the categories listed below and on the next page. Write at least two specific interventions for each category that should be part of David Ruskin's care while he remains in the hospital.

Category	Interventions
Promoting effective breathing	
Promoting effective coughing	

Category	Interventions
Promoting activity	
Promoting comfort	
Maintaining fluid and electrolyte balance	
Relieving abdominal distention	
Promoting tissue perfusion	
Promoting urinary elimination	
Preventing injury	
Preventing wound infection	
Patient and family education	

LESSON **12** ─────────────────────

Chronic Obstructive Pulmonary Disease

 Reading Assignment: Assessment of the Respiratory System (Chapter 19)
Lower Airway Problems (Chapter 21)

Patient: Sally Begay, Room 304

In this lesson you will focus on chronic obstructive pulmonary disease (COPD) by exploring the respiratory history of Sally Begay, a 58-year-old Navajo woman. Have a drug reference book available for use if needed during this lesson.

Writing Activity

1. It is essential to take a current health history to properly evaluate a respiratory disorder. For each of the common respiratory complaints listed below and on the next page, write two questions that could be used to further evaluate each symptom. *Hint:* Use information in the Health History section on pp. 461–464 of the textbook if needed.

Respiratory Symptom	Sample Questions to Evaluate the Symptom
Dyspnea	
Cough	
Sputum production	
Hemoptysis	

Respiratory Symptom	**Sample Questions to Evaluate the Symptom**
Wheezing	
Chest pain	
Upper respiratory symptoms	

2. Identify specific data to gather about the timing and characteristics of dyspnea when conducting a symptom analysis of this condition.

Timing

Characteristics

📀 CD-ROM Activity

Go to the Supervisor's Office and sign in to work with Sally Begay at 0700 on Tuesday. Next, go to the Nurses' Station and open her chart. In the History and Physical section, read the admitting history completed on Saturday at 1200 in the emergency department. As you read, consider questions 3–5.

3. For how long has Sally Begay had bronchitis?

4. In addition to the respiratory diagnoses of pneumonia and COPD, what other types of medical diagnoses does Sally Begay have?

5. Listed below are the prescribed and over-the-counter medications Sally Begay is taking. For each medication, identify the classification and reason she is taking it.

Medication Name and Dose	Classification and Reason for Taking
HCTZ 25 mg QD	
Digoxin 0.125 mg QD	
NTG grains 1/150 SL PRN	
Acetaminophen 650 mg q4h PRN	
Pseudoephedrine 30 mg 3–4x/day	
"Some type of nose spray"	

In your textbook, read the sections describing chronic obstructive pulmonary disease, emphysema, and chronic bronchitis (pp. 566–569).

6. Define the following terms.

Chronic obstructive pulmonary disease (COPD)

Emphysema

Chronic bronchitis

7. List four risk factors in the etiology of COPD. Circle the leading risk factor.

   a.

   b.

   c.

   d.

8. Based on the history that you read in Sally Begay's chart, identify the etiology(ies) most likely to be responsible for her COPD.

9. Summarize briefly the pathophysiology of chronic bronchitis.

10. What relationship is there between Sally Begay's admitting diagnosis of pneumonia and her underlying condition of chronic bronchitis?

➡ Now return to the chart to review the results of the chest x-ray that was ordered for Sally Begay. To do this, click on **Diagnostics** and read the radiological report by Dr. Kawasaka.

11. What findings listed in the chest x-ray report are consistent with COPD? *Hint:* The general discussion of chest x-ray studies in Chapter 19 of the textbook may be helpful in understanding the results.

➡ To gather data for question 12, first return to the History and Physical in Sally Begay's chart and find the vital signs taken in the ED on Saturday. Next, access the EPR and click on **Blood Gases**. Find Sally Begay's oxygen saturation results for Saturday at 1600 and 2000.

12. a. In the middle column below, record the O_2 saturation results you found in Sally Begay's chart and EPR. Record the normal range in the third column.

Medical Record Documentation	Sally Begay's O_2 Saturation	Normal Range for O_2 Saturation
Emergency department report at 1200		
ABGs at 1600		
ABGs at 2000		

b. Review Sally Begay's O_2 saturation values above. What conclusion can you make about her progress based on these values?

13. What does the arterial oxygen saturation (SaO_2) reflect? Why does Sally Begay's level not fall within the normal range?

➡ Next click on **Physicians' Orders**. Review the orders written on Sunday night.

14. What order was written for oxygen therapy? What percentage of oxygen does this deliver? *Hint:* Refer to Table 21-3 on textbook p. 531 if needed.

15. What makes this oxygen order preferable to high-flow oxygen administration to relieve the hypoxia Sally Begay is experiencing?

16. What medication is specifically ordered for treatment of COPD? How does the drug work? How should it be administered? *Hint:* Refer to a drug handbook and to Table 21-11 on textbook p. 571 if needed.

➡ Click on **Nurses' Notes** and read the note for Saturday at 2100.

17. What problems did the nurse identify? What interventions are planned? How should the effectiveness of the interventions be evaluated? Write your answers in the table below and on the next page.

Identified Problems	Planned Interventions	Evaluation Methods

Identified Problems	Planned Interventions	Evaluation Methods

18. Compare the problems and planned interventions from the Nurses' Notes with the nursing diagnoses listed on p. 575 of the textbook. Based on what you know so far about Sally Begay, what additional nursing diagnoses should be added to her problem list?

→ Return to Sally Begay's EPR. Click on **Vital Signs** and **Assessments** to answer question 19.

19. Below, record the nursing assessment data documented in Sally Begay's EPR on Saturday at 1600 and Tuesday at 0400.

Assessment Areas	Saturday 1600	Tuesday 0400
Temperature		
Heart rate		
Respiration		
Oxygen saturation		
Use of oxygen		
Respiratory pattern		
Lung fields		
Cough		
Sputum		

20. Based on your findings in question 19, evaluate whether Sally Begay's condition has improved since Saturday. How successful have the interventions been to date? What additional information do you need to consider?

21. What additional interventions may be helpful at this point in time? *Hint:* Consider information on pp. 577–579 of the textbook if needed.

➤ You have completed your assignment for Tuesday. Go back to the Supervisor's Office and sign in for Thursday at 1100, keeping Sally Begay as your patient. After you sign in, you hear from the other nurses that she is approaching the time of discharge. It is your priority to be involved with her discharge planning, so go directly to the Nurses' Station and find the location for the health team meeting. Attend the meeting and take notes for question 22 below as you listen.

22. Below, record important discharge data addressed by each of the health team members.

Person Reporting	Important Discharge Planning Data
Rose Simpson, RN Case manager	
Louise Johnson, RN Clinical nurse specialist	
Kris Holmes, MSW Social worker	

23. Reflect on the information you just heard in the health team report. Compare the data you recorded in question 22 with the information in your textbook on pp. 577–579. What additional considerations for discharge planning would you like to include in a teaching plan for this patient?

24. When teaching Sally Begay about health promotion and prevention of respiratory disease, what two vaccines should be included in the discussion? *Hint:* Refer to Health Promotion/Prevention on textbook p. 579 if needed.

LESSON 13 _____

Pneumonia, Part 1

/OᴅᴏO **Reading Assignment:** Assessment of the Respiratory System (Chapter 19)
Lower Airway Problems (Chapter 21)

Patient: Sally Begay, Room 304

In this lesson, you will complete a preclinical record review in preparation for caring for Sally Begay, a 58-year-old Navajo woman who has been admitted with a diagnosis of pneumonia. She has an underlying history of mild COPD, which was the focus of the previous lesson. Be sure to have a laboratory and diagnostic test reference book available as you complete this lesson.

CD-ROM Activity

Go to the Supervisor's Office and sign in to work with Sally Begay for Tuesday at 0700. Next, go to the Nurses' Station and open her chart. Click on **History and Physical** and read the admitting report done in the emergency department on Saturday at 1200. Use information from this record to answer questions 1–3.

1. What is Sally Begay's admitting diagnosis?

2. What are her primary symptoms, and for how long has she had them? *Hint:* Scroll down to find this information in the History of Present Illness section of the chart.

3. What other health problems are documented in Sally Begay's history? *Hint:* Look in the Significant Medical History section.

115

Originally, a suspected diagnosis for Sally Begay was Hantavirus infection, which is a less common health problem that is not often discussed in nursing textbooks. You decide to investigate this illness on the hospital Intranet. Close the chart and access the Intranet on the computer to the left of the chart shelf in the Nurses' Station. Gather information to answer questions 4 and 5 by reviewing the CDC website at http://www.cdc.gov/ncidod/diseases/hanta/hps/noframes/othrsrce.htm.

4. What is Hantavirus?

5. Based on what you have learned about Hantavirus and what you have read in Sally Begay's chart, make one list below of data supporting a diagnosis of Hantavirus and another list supporting a diagnosis of pneumonia.

Hantavirus   **Pneumonia**

 6. The final diagnosis for Sally Begay is pneumonia. How does your textbook define *pneumonia*? *Hint:* Discussion of pneumonia begins on p. 525 in your textbook.

7. Identify from your textbook the major etiologies of pneumonia.

8. Because Sally Begay has been hospitalized, she may also be at risk for developing hospital-acquired pneumonia (HAP). The risk factors for HAP are listed below. Place a check mark next to each risk factor that applies to Sally Begay.

Risk Factors for Hospital Acquired Pneumonia	Applies to Sally Begay
Treatment in an intensive care unit (ICU)	_____
Mechanical ventilation	_____
Endotracheal intubation or tracheostomy	_____
Recent surgery	_____
Debilitation or malnutrition	_____
Invasive devices	_____
Neuromuscular disease	_____
Depressed level of alertness	_____
Aspiration	_____
Antacid use	_____
Age 60 or older	_____
Prolonged hospital stay	_____
Any serious underlying disease	_____

9. Which chronic disease state found in Sally Begay's medical history is the one that most likely contributed directly to development of pneumonia? Briefly explain your answer.

➡ Return to Sally Begay's chart and click on **Physicians' Orders**. Read the first set of orders written on Saturday at 1230.

📖 10. Compare the diagnostic tests ordered with the ones identified in your textbook on p. 1713. Place a check mark next to the diagnostic tests that were ordered for Sally Begay.

_____ Chest x-ray

_____ Sputum culture, sensitivity, and Gram stain

_____ Fiberoptic bronchoscopy

_____ White blood cell count

_____ Blood cultures

_____ Cold agglutinins

_____ Arterial blood gas measurements

_____ Thoracentesis

➡ Now click on **Diagnostics** to check the availability of results for the diagnostic tests that were ordered.

11. What findings in the chest x-ray report support the diagnosis of pneumonia? *Hint:* The description of expected chest x-ray findings is on p. 527 in your textbook.

12. What do the other chest x-ray findings suggest?

13. The textbook identifies the following clinical manifestations associated with the onset of community-acquired pneumonia. Place a check mark next to each manifestation exhibited by Sally Begay. *Hint:* Return to the History and Physical in her chart if needed.

_____   Fever

_____   Rigors (chills accompanied by shaking)

_____   Sweats

_____   Cough

_____   Sputum production

_____   Change in color of sputum

_____   Chest discomfort

_____   Dyspnea

→ Close the chart and access Sally Begay's EPR. Click on **Hematology** and find the laboratory results for the CBC that was completed on Saturday.

14. For each lab test listed below, record Sally Begay's results from the EPR, as well as the normal reference range for that test. Place an asterisk next to any abnormal result. *Hint:* You may need to consult a laboratory and diagnostic test reference book to obtain this information.

Laboratory Test	Sally Begay's Result	Normal Reference Range
Hemoglobin (Hgb)		
Hematocrit (Hct)		
White blood cell (WBC) count		
Red blood cell (RBC) count		
Platelets		

15. What is the significance of the abnormal values you found in question 14, if any?

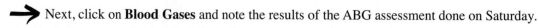 Next, click on **Blood Gases** and note the results of the ABG assessment done on Saturday.

16. For each blood gas component listed below, record Sally Begay's results for Saturday, as well as the normal reference range for that test. Place an asterisk next to any abnormal result. *Hint:* Refer to Table 19-8 on p. 471 of your textbook or a laboratory reference book if you need help interpreting blood gas results.

Blood Gas Component	Sally Begay's Result	Normal Reference Range
pH		
$PaCO_2$		
PaO_2		
HCO_3^-		
O_2 saturation		

17. What is the significance of the arterial blood gas results recorded in question 16?

→ Next, review the assessment data gathered for Sally Begay's Admissions Profile. Click on **Admissions** in the EPR and scroll through the information documented there. Take notes below of any data that relate to the respiratory system. (You will use these data later when formulating a plan of nursing care.)

Student Notes

→ Now click on **Assessments** and find the most recent data collected on Tuesday at 0400. Record your findings below. (This will provide you with baseline data for the assessment you will conduct in the next lesson.)

18.   **Tuesday 0400 Findings**

Chest expansion

Nailbeds

Respiratory pattern

Lung fields

Cough

Sputum

→ Close the EPR and open the MAR in the blue notebook on the counter. Review the medications ordered for Sally Begay for today.

19. For each time listed below, list the medication(s) to be given and the reason for administration.

Time	Scheduled Medication(s)	Reason for Giving
0900		
1200		
1400		

20. You have gathered a sufficient background database to begin to formulate a plan of care for Sally Begay. Use this database and the information on textbook pp. 529–532 to begin your care planning below.

Nursing Diagnoses	Outcomes	Interventions

LESSON 14

Pneumonia, Part 2

👓 **Reading Assignment:** Lower Airway Problems (Chapter 21)

Patient: Sally Begay, Room 304

In this lesson you will implement care for Sally Begay, a 58-year-old Navajo woman admitted with pneumonia. If you have not complete Lesson 13, do so before beginning this lesson. Be sure to have a drug reference book available to use as a reference during your shift.

💿 **CD-ROM Activity**

Go to the Supervisor's Office and sign in to work with Sally Begay on Thursday at 0700. Next, go to the Nurses' Station and look on the bulletin board to find the location of the intershift report for this patient. Go there and listen to the report on Sally Begay. As you listen, fill in answers to question 1 on the next page or take notes below and use your notes to complete question 1.

Student Notes

---

1. Complete the following report sheet to use as reference during your shift.

Patient:	Room #:
Age:	Diagnosis:

Vital signs:

O₂ sat:	Pain:

Treatments:

Significant assessment findings:

IV location/date:

Identified patient/family problems:

Items requiring follow-up:

2. What piece of information was stated in error during intershift report?

➤ It will be a busy morning now that Sally Begay is scheduled for discharge. You decide to measure vital signs to begin the day's work. Go to her room and click on **Vital Signs**.

3. Measure Sally Begay's vital signs and record your findings below.

Blood pressure _____   Heart rate _____   Oxygen saturation _____

Temperature _____   Respiratory rate _____   Pain rating _____

4. What did you observe during the oxygen saturation measurement that could affect the accuracy of the reading?

5. Review the vital signs that you recorded in question 3. Are they within normal range? Are they satisfactory given that Sally Begay will be discharged this morning? Review your notes from report as you answer this question.

➤ While you are still in Sally Begay's room, complete a physical examination. Click first on **Physical** and then on each of the three examination areas, one at a time.

6. Below, record your data for each area in the physical examination.

Physical Examination Area	Data Obtained
Head and Neck	

Physical Examination Area	Data Obtained
Chest/Upper Extremities	
Abdomen and Lower Extremities	

7. What data are useful in determining Sally Begay's readiness for discharge? Do you have any concerns at this time, given the information you have obtained?

➤ Return to the Nurses' Station and access Sally Begay's EPR. First, click on **Vital Signs** and chart your findings from question 3. Next click on **Assessments** and chart the findings from question 6. You are now ready to administer medications to Sally Begay. Open the MAR and note what medications are scheduled during your shift today; use this data to answer question 8. Once you are finished, return to Sally Begay's room and administer her medications.

8. Below and on the next page, record the medications that are due for Sally Begay between 0700 and 1500 today. For each medication, include the time and reason to be given.

Time	Scheduled Medication	Reason for Giving Medication

Time	Scheduled Medication	Reason for Giving Medication

9. What two medications have monitoring parameters assigned to them? Can they safely be given to Sally Begay at this time?

10. Ceftizoxime is ordered to be given by the IVPB route. The IV solution running in the primary IV line is $D_5 \frac{1}{2}$ NS. Are these two solutions compatible? How will you determine this?

11. Sally Begay has been taking oral fluids. Why does she still have an IV running at 75 ml/hour?

12. What medication was written as being discontinued in the Stat/Pre-op/One Time area? How would you verify that this is correct?

➤ Return to Sally Begay's chart, click on **Physicians' Orders**, and review the newest set of orders written at 0630.

13. What three new orders were written by the physician at 0630?

   a.

   b.

   c.

14. Use your clinical reasoning skills to draw one conclusion about each of the orders written in Question 13. Draw on all the information you have gathered for this patient thus far as you exercise your clinical judgment.

➤ Return to Sally Begay's room and administer the medications ordered for 0900. Let her rest for a short period of time while you prepare your discharge instructions. Even though the physician has postponed discharge until Friday, you know it is important to allow sufficient time for teaching and learning in order to support a smooth transition from hospital to home and to promote optimal health after discharge.

15. Develop a teaching plan that will help Sally Begay to avoid readmission for this health problem. *Hint:* Refer to pp. 530–531 of your textbook for suggestions.

Coronary Artery Disease

 Reading Assignment: Assessment of the Cardiovascular System (Chapter 22)
Dysrhythmias and Coronary Artery Disease (Chapter 23)

Patient: Sally Begay, Room 304

In this lesson you will have an opportunity to do a record review and a patient assessment to learn more about coronary artery disease. You will be working with Sally Begay, the 58-year-old Navajo woman admitted with a diagnosis of pneumonia and a history of hypertension, coronary heart disease, and myocardial infarction. It may be helpful to have a drug reference book and a nutrition textbook available for reference during this lesson.

Writing Activity

1. Identify and describe six important clinical manifestations to inquire about when obtaining a health history to determine risk for cardiac disease. *Hint:* use information on pp. 624–625 if needed.

2. Sally Begay is a member of the Navajo American Indian tribe. What role does race play in the development of coronary artery disease according to the textbook?

CD-ROM Activity

Go to the Supervisor's Office and sign in to work with Sally Begay on Thursday at 0700. Go to the Nurses' Station and open her chart. Click on **History and Physical** and read the complete admission history taken on Saturday at 1200. Use questions 3 and 4 to guide your reading.

3. Consider the following risk factors for cardiovascular disease as presented in the textbook. Next to each risk factor, check "Yes" if it applies to Sally Begay, "No" if it does not, and "NA" if the information is not available. When you are done, review the list of risk factors checked "Yes," and circle those that can be modified by Ms. Begay if she chooses.

Risk Factor	Yes	No	NA
Age and gender	_____	_____	_____
Family history	_____	_____	_____
Diabetes	_____	_____	_____
Hypertension	_____	_____	_____
Tobacco use	_____	_____	_____
Sedentary lifestyle	_____	_____	_____
Dyslipidemia	_____	_____	_____
Obesity	_____	_____	_____
Diet	_____	_____	_____
Stress	_____	_____	_____

4. Continue reviewing the History and Physical in Sally Begay's chart, recording data related to each of the clinical manifestations of heart disease listed below. If no documentation is provided about an item, write "None."

Chest pain

Palpitations

Dyspnea

Syncope

Fatigue

Weight gain/dependent edema

5. The medical record clearly indicates that Sally Begay is experiencing pain in her chest. How might you differentiate chest pain of cardiac origin from the chest pain she is experiencing because of pneumonia? *Hint:* Refer to p. 651 in the textbook.

Close Sally Begay's chart and access her EPR. Click on **Admissions** and read her list of current medications in the section "Support Network/Self-Care." Note also her answers to the questions in the section "Sleep and Relaxation"; then answer the questions below. Use a drug reference book if needed.

6. Record the name and dose of each medication Sally Begay is taking, the drug category to which it belongs, and the reason why she is taking it. (Infer the reasons from what you have read in the chart and the information in your drug handbook).

Medication Name and Dose	Drug Category	Reason for Taking

7. Why would it also be important to ask Sally Begay about the type(s) of tea she drinks to relax?

 Chapter 23 identifies three somewhat overlapping coronary syndromes: stable angina, acute coronary syndrome, and myocardial infarction. Review the information about angina and myocardial infarction if needed; then answer the following questions.

8. Sally Begay's significant medical history lists "MI five years ago, mild CHF, and stable angina" in the section on heart disease in the History and Physical. What is angina?

9. Describe what occurs during an episode of angina. *Hint:* See pp. 647–648 of the textbook.

10. According to Sally Begay's history, how frequently does she experience chest pain?

11. The following electrocardiographic tracings are associated with myocardial ischemia. For each tracing, label the alteration that is occurring in that ECG complex. *Hint:* Refer to Figure 23-7 on p. 652 of your textbook if needed.

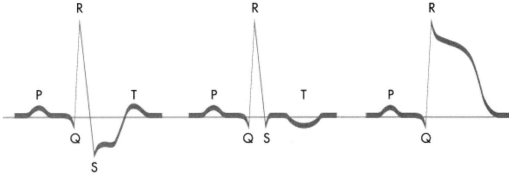

a. _____   b. _____   c. _____

 12. Look back at the medications you identified in question 6. Which of these was ordered in case Sally Begay had an episode of angina? How does this medication work to treat angina? *Hint:* Use your drug handbook or Table 23-5 in your textbook as a guide.

13. Sally Begay had a myocardial infarction (MI) 5 years ago. What is an MI, and what happens during the process?

14. What relationship, if any, is there between hypertension and experiencing a myocardial infarction?

15. How can a myocardial infarction subsequently lead to development of heart failure?

➤ Now take your own health history of Sally Begay in preparation for developing an individualized teaching plan for angina pectoris. Go to her room and click on **Health History**. Then, one at a time, click on **Culture**, **Activity**, and **Nutrition-Metabolic**.

16. As you listen to Sally Begay's health history in each of these areas, take notes below about pertinent information that will help you develop your teaching plan.

Culture

Activity

Nutrition-Metabolic

17. Use the information you gathered in question 16 to formulate an individualized teaching plan for Sally Begay about ways to minimize angina attacks. To organize your plan, use the framework identified on textbook p. 674 in the Patient Teaching: The Patient with Coronary Artery Disease box. Develop your teaching plan below.

Risk Factor Modification

Resumption of Activity

Medications

LESSON 16

Heart Failure Part 1

Reading Assignment: Assessment of the Cardiovascular System (Chapter 22)
Heart Failure, Valvular Problems, and Inflammatory Problems
of the Heart (Chapter 24)

Patient: Carmen Gonzales, Room 302

In this lesson you will work with Carmen Gonzales, a 56-year-old woman admitted for treatment of an infected left lower leg wound. Her significant history includes type 2 diabetes mellitus (DM), hypertension, coronary artery disease (CAD), and heart failure.

 Writing Activity

To fully understand heart failure, you must comprehend how the heart normally functions as a pump. Match each of the following terms related to normal cardiac physiology with its definition. *Hint:* Use the information on textbook pp. 617–620 or a medical dictionary if needed.

	Term	Definition
1. _____	Afterload	a. Positive inotropism that improves stroke volume.
2. _____	Cardiac output	b. The resistance to left ventricular ejection.
3. _____	Diastole	c. The volume of blood ejected with each contraction of the ventricle.
4. _____	Contractility	
5. _____	Heart rate	d. The amount of blood ejected per minute by the ventricles, usually 4–8 liters/minute.
6. _____	Preload	e. The myocardial fiber length at end diastole.
7. _____	Stroke volume	f. The number of cardiac contractions/minute.
8. _____	Systole	g. The phase of the cardiac cycle characterized by relaxation and filling of the atria or ventricles.
		h. The phase of the cardiac cycle characterized by contraction and emptying of the atria or ventricles.

9. How is cardiac output determined using stroke volume and heart rate?

10. Review what you have just read about the concepts of preload, afterload, and contractility. Describe the effect of each of these concepts on the stroke volume pumped by the heart.

How preload affects stroke volume:

How afterload affects stroke volume:

How contractility affects stroke volume:

CD-ROM Activity

Go to the Supervisor's Office and sign in to work with Carmen Gonzales on Tuesday at 0700. Next, go to the Nurses' Station and open her chart. Click on **History and Physical** and read the entire report, including the Emergency Department Record. Search for any information that addresses heart failure or risk for heart failure.

11. What information did you find in the History section and in the Physical Examination section of the chart that addresses Carmen Gonzales' status in relation to heart failure?

History section

Physical Examination section

 12. If you had conducted the initial assessment in the emergency department, would you have gathered any additional assessment data (history or physical examination) related to heart failure? If so, what? *Hint:* Refer to Clinical Manifestations on pp. 716–718 in your textbook if needed.

13. Several events can affect the development of heart failure in a patient. Review the copy of Box 24-6 below and place a check mark next to each factor that is likely an etiology of heart failure for Carmen Gonzales.

Precipitating Events in Decompensated Heart Failure

Factors Increasing Myocardial Demand
Additional Increases in Ventricular Volume to Be Pumped
Hypervolemia from high-output states (e.g., pregnancy, anemia, hyperthyroidism, infection)
Aortic regurgitation
Mitral regurgitation
Excessive sodium intake
Excessive administration of fluids
Renal failure

An Increase in the Ventricular Force Needed to Eject Blood
Poorly controlled systemic hypertension
Pulmonary hypertension
Significant aortic stenosis
Significant pulmonic stenosis

Factors Interfering with the Heart's Ability to Contract or Fill
Myocardial ischemia
Myocardial infarction
Cardiomyopathy
Myocarditis
Ventricular aneurysm
Excess alcohol intake
Cardiac tamponade
Restrictive pericarditis
Dysrhythmias

---

14. Based on what you have learned thus far about Carmen Gonzales, identify two specific triggers that are likely to have precipitated temporary decompensation of her status with regard to heart failure.

 It is time to listen to report on Carmen Gonzales. Close the chart and check the bulletin board for the report location. Go to the appropriate room and listen to the report. As you are listening, take notes below of any information related to potential or actual heart failure.

Student Notes

15. Reflect on the information you heard in the report. Are there other data you wish the nurse had included related to heart failure? Explain. The night nurse suggested you keep a "close eye" on Carmen Gonzales. What will you look for?

→ To seek more information about Carmen Gonzales' condition in relation to heart failure, access her EPR, click on **Admissions**, and read the Admissions Profile.

16. What information in Carmen Gonzales' profile gives you additional clues about the presence of symptoms of heart failure?

→ Now click on **I&O** and review Carmen Gonzales' intake and output patterns from Sunday at 2400 until Tuesday at 0800. Note her fluid balance trend by answering the following questions.

17. What was Carmen Gonzales' net fluid balance at each of the following times?

Sunday 2400 _____   Monday 1200 _____   Monday 2400 _____

Monday 0400 _____   Monday 1600 _____   Tuesday 0400 _____

Monday 0800 _____   Monday 2000 _____   Tuesday 0800 _____

18. Add the numbers you wrote in question 17 above to determine Carmen Gonzales' overall fluid balance. Record it below.

19. How much of a weight change should be expected in Carmen Gonzales over this time period based on changes in her body fluid balance? Calculate this number after recalling that 1 liter of fluid equals approximately 1 kilogram, or 2.2 pounds.

→ Close the EPR and return to the chart one more time before going to assess Carmen Gonzales. Click on **Physicians' Orders** and review the written orders.

20. Which orders are written for Carmen Gonzales that specifically relate to assessing for and treating heart failure?

➡ Now go to Carmen Gonzales' room and click on **Vital Signs**.

21. Measure her vital signs for 0800 and record them below.

Blood pressure _____ Heart rate _____ Oxygen saturation _____

Temperature _____ Respiratory rate _____ Pain rating _____

➡ Next, conduct a physical assessment of Carmen Gonzales so that you can develop a plan of care. Click on **Physical**; then (one at a time) click on **Head and Neck**, **Chest/Upper Extremities**, and **Abdomen and Lower Extremities**. As you conduct the examination, fill in question 22 below.

22. Record any data, either normal or abnormal, that provide useful information about the presence or absence of heart failure.

	Normal Data	Abnormal Data
Head and Neck		
Chest/Upper Extremities		
Abdomen and Lower Extremities		

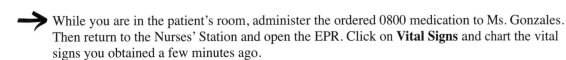 While you are in the patient's room, administer the ordered 0800 medication to Ms. Gonzales. Then return to the Nurses' Station and open the EPR. Click on **Vital Signs** and chart the vital signs you obtained a few minutes ago.

23. Review the vital signs you obtained in question 21. Do any of the results concern you, and if so, which one(s) and why?

24. Now that you have charted Carmen Gonzales' 0800 vital signs in the EPR, compare those readings with the ones taken over the last few days. What would be an appropriate action to take at this time?

 25. Consider the entire database you have gathered to this point. Use your clinical diagnostic reasoning skills to determine a list of actual or risk nursing diagnoses. If you need cuing, refer to p. 725 of your textbook or another nursing diagnosis reference book. Don't forget to include a diagnosis that would consider teaching/learning needs.

LESSON 17

Heart Failure
Part 2

/OO **Reading Assignment:** Heart Failure, Valvular Problems, and Inflammatory Problems of
the Heart (Chapter 24)

Patient: Carmen Gonzales, Room 302

In this lesson you continue to care for Carmen Gonzales, a 56-year-old woman admitted for
treatment of an infected left lower leg wound. Her significant history includes diabetes mellitus
type 2, hypertension, coronary heart disease, and heart failure. If you have not completed
Lesson 16, do so prior to beginning this lesson. You should also have a drug reference book and
a nutrition textbook available to help you answer some of the questions in this lesson.

CD-ROM Activity

Go to the Supervisor's Office and sign in to work with Carmen Gonzales at 0700 on Thursday.
Proceed to the Nurses' Station and click on the bulletin board to find the location of report on
Ms. Gonzales. Go to hear the report, taking notes below related to heart failure. This will provide a basis for your care today. If you are unsure of what manifestations are relevant, review
your textbook or refer back to your notes from the previous lesson.

Student Notes

145

→ After report, return to the Nurses' Station, open Carmen Gonzales' chart, and look for additional information about changes in her condition since Tuesday morning, when you cared for her last. Specifically, click on **Nurses' Notes** and review documentation for Tuesday afternoon and Wednesday. Note any significant data related to heart failure.

1. Identify any significant information in the nurses' notes related to heart failure.

→ Next, click on **Physicians' Notes** and read the cardiology consult written Tuesday afternoon at 1505.

2. What data were recorded in this note related to heart failure?

→ Click on **Physicians' Orders** and read the orders written Tuesday at 1515.

3. Record the orders written on Tuesday afternoon that relate to exacerbation of heart failure.

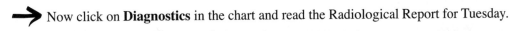 Now click on **Diagnostics** in the chart and read the Radiological Report for Tuesday.

    4. What is your interpretation of the Tuesday afternoon chest x-ray results? Explain.

    5. According to the chart, what type of heart failure did Carmen Gonzales experience on Tuesday afternoon? What was the precipitating factor? Would this be characterized as acute failure or chronic failure? Why?

     6. Identify the clinical manifestations of heart failure exhibited by Carmen Gonzales. Using the descriptions provided in Box 24-5 of the textbook, are these signs more consistent with left-sided heart failure or right-sided heart failure? What other signs would you look for that are not documented in the medical record?

Close Carmen Gonzales' chart and access her EPR. Click on **I&O** to determine her fluid balance. (You completed a similar exercise in Lesson 16 using a different method of calculation.)

7. Below, record Carmen Gonzales' I&O records since admission. Then, calculate 3-day totals for her input and output.

	Total Intake	Total Output
Sunday		
Monday		
Tuesday until 1200		
3-Day totals		

 Writing Activity

8. Consider the data you collected in question 7 above and draw conclusions about Carmen Gonzales' fluid balance. What nursing actions could have and should have been taken to prevent this situation from occurring or to limit its severity? Form a conclusion about the quality of this aspect of nursing care.

 9. Reflect on your knowledge of the pathophysiologic basis for the clinical manifestations of heart failure as explained in your textbook. How did fluid overload contribute to the development of her signs and symptoms? What type of medication therapy do you anticipate being ordered?

Refer back to your answer to question 3 to see what medication the physician ordered for Ms. Gonzales on Tuesday. Use your drug reference book and Table 24-3 in the textbook to answer questions 10 through 12.

10. What is the mechanism of action of this medication? Where and how does it work?

11. What will you look for as the therapeutic effect? How will you know that this effect has been achieved?

12. Why is this medication a better drug of choice than another medication in the same general class? For what reason was it given by the IV route for the first dose, before ordering it as an oral medication?

13. Below, note the change in I&O records after Carmen Gonzales received the ordered medication. *Hint:* Get the 3-day totals from your answers to question 7.

	Total Intake	Total Output
3-day totals from question 7		
Sunday–Tuesday 1200		
Tuesday 1600–2400		
Wednesday		
Thursday until 0800		
New cumulative totals		

14. What conclusions can you draw from the data you recorded in question 13?

 Knowing that fluid and electrolyte balance often go hand-in-hand, you decide to check Carmen Gonzales' electrolyte levels drawn Tuesday evening (as part of the "Chem 7" order) and correlate them with the values noted on an earlier lab draw. While you still have access to the EPR, click on **Chemistry** and note the electrolyte results on Tuesday at 0800 before the episode of heart failure and on Tuesday at 2000 after the episode. Then answer questions 15 and 16.

15. Record Carmen Gonzales' sodium and potassium levels in the spaces below.

	Tuesday 0800	Tuesday 2000
Sodium		
Potassium		

16. Did the values for these major electrolytes change in the direction(s) that you expected? Explain.

→ Close the EPR and open the blue MAR on the counter across from the chart shelf. Access Carmen Gonzales' record and review the medications scheduled for the day.

17. You are working today from 0700 to 1500. Write down the medications you will administer to Carmen Gonzales during that period, along with the time each drug is due, and a reminder note to yourself about the reason she is getting each medication.

Medication	Time Due	Reason for Taking

→ It is time to measure vital signs and administer 0800 medications to Carmen Gonzales. Go to her room and click on **Vital Signs**.

18. Obtain a set of vital signs and record your findings below.

Blood pressure _____   Heart rate _____   Oxygen saturation _____

Temperature _____   Respiratory rate _____   Pain rating _____

→ Give Carmen Gonzales the ordered medications while you are still in her room, especially since her breakfast tray has just arrived. Once you are finished, return to her EPR, click on **Vital Signs**, and chart her 0800 vital signs in the proper area. Note how her current vital signs compare with previous readings.

As part of the plan of care for today, you need to participate in discharge planning and patient teaching for Carmen Gonzales. To accomplish this, you will need to do several things. Close the EPR and look on the bulletin board for the location of the health team meeting. Go to the meeting and listen to the reports of each of the health team members. Then find the patient's chart and click on **Health Team**. Read this report and review the following to refresh your memory as needed:
- The History and Physical in the chart
- The health history interview and physical examination data you obtained on Tuesday
- The Admissions Profile in the EPR

19. What particular issues will you keep in mind as you approach discharge teaching, given the specific issues identified in the data for Carmen Gonzales?

20. How will culture influence the discharge teaching you conduct with Ms. Gonzales?

21. Using a nutrition book, complete a teaching plan for Carmen Gonzales about a low-sodium diet by answering the questions below and on the next page.

   a. What is a low-sodium diet?

   b. Why is this type of diet important as part of treatment for heart failure?

c. What foods can Ms. Gonzales enjoy while following a low-sodium diet?

d. List some examples of foods Ms. Gonzales should avoid while she is on this diet.

 22. After you complete teaching Carmen Gonzales about a low-sodium diet, you consider other aspects of her discharge teaching plan. Refer to the Patient Teaching: Heart Failure box on textbook p. 728 and write a teaching plan that is modified to meet the needs of Carmen Gonzales.

Hypertension

📖 **Reading Assignment:** Assessment of the Cardiovascular System (Chapter 22)
Vascular Problems (Chapter 25)

Patient: Sally Begay, Room 304

In this lesson you will learn about hypertension by exploring the history of Sally Begay, a 58-year-old Navajo woman admitted with pneumonia. Her pertinent history includes chronic bronchitis, coronary artery disease, and a myocardial infarction 5 years ago.

📘 In your textbook, review the cardiac cycle and the anatomy and physiology of the peripheral vascular system on pp. 620–624 of the textbook, as well as the pathophysiology of hypertension on pp. 760–761. Then answer the following questions.

✒️ **Writing Activity**

1. In your own words, describe the concept of blood pressure.

2. What are the two mechanisms that provide overall control of blood pressure?

3. Briefly explain each of the blood pressure control mechanisms you identified in question 2. *Hint:* Refer to textbook pp. 760–761.

CD-ROM Activity

Go to the Supervisor's Office and sign in to work with Sally Begay for Thursday at 1100. Next, go to the Nurses' Station and open her chart. Click on **History and Physical**, and read the admission history completed Saturday at 1200. Use questions 4 through 7 as a focus for your reading.

4. For how long has Sally Begay had a history of hypertension?

5. What was her blood pressure (BP) when she was seen in the emergency department?

6. What manifestations is she likely to experience when her BP reaches that level?

7. What pharmacologic agents does Ms. Begay currently take at home according to the Current Medication section of her chart? Write the name and dose of each medication below, and indicate the classification of each medication in parentheses. Which of these drugs was ordered for hypertension?

8. How is the term *hypertension* defined in your textbook?

9. What is the difference between *primary hypertension* and *secondary hypertension*?

Primary hypertension

Secondary hypertension

10. From what you have read in Sally Begay's chart so far, do you think she has primary hypertension or secondary hypertension? Give a brief rationale for your answer.

➤ Close Sally Begay's chart and open her EPR. Click on **Admissions** and read her entire Admissions Profile. Use questions 11 and 12 to help focus your reading.

11. Based on the data in her Admissions Profile and the Emergency Department Report in her chart, what nonmodifiable and modifiable risk factors does Sally Begay have?

12. The Admissions Profile contains several pieces of information that may help to indicate how Sally Begay manages her blood pressure while she is at home. What are they, and what significance do they have?

13. When blood pressure rises sufficiently, clinical manifestations become apparent. What are the manifestations that provide a clue that a patient may have severely elevated blood pressure?

14. Consider again Sally Begay's blood pressure upon presentation to the Emergency Department. (Look back to your answer to question 5 if needed). In what classification or category would you place Sally Begay's blood pressure? Why? *Hint:* Use Table 25-2 if needed.

15. Review the information in your textbook presented in Table 25-3: Risk Stratification and Treatment of Hypertension. To what risk group does Sally Begay belong, based on her admission blood pressure? Why?

16. Explain the purpose of risk stratification. How does this impact the treatment that Sally Begay receives?

⟶ Close the EPR and open Sally Begay's chart. This time click on **Physicians' Orders** and read her admission orders.

17. Note that the diagnostic tests and lab tests listed below and on the next page were ordered to provide evidence of target organ damage from hypertension. Describe how each test is useful in determining the presence of target organ damage.

Chest x-ray

ECG monitoring

BUN

Creatinine

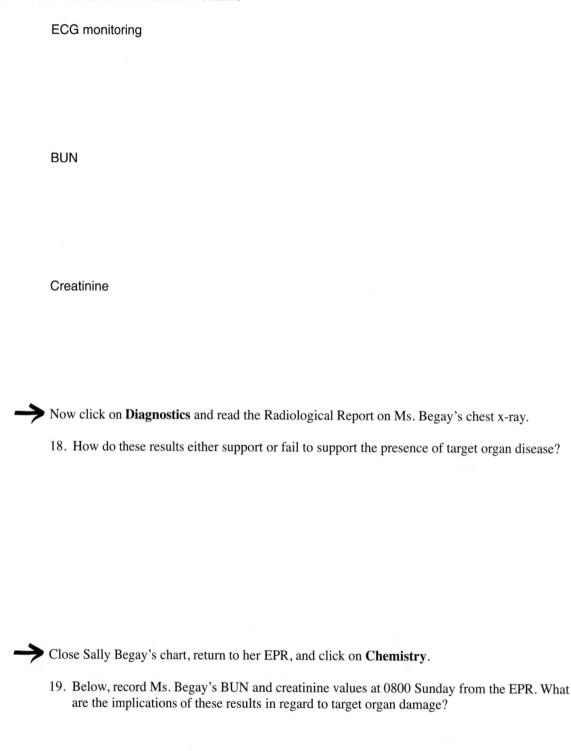 Now click on **Diagnostics** and read the Radiological Report on Ms. Begay's chest x-ray.

18. How do these results either support or fail to support the presence of target organ disease?

Close Sally Begay's chart, return to her EPR, and click on **Chemistry**.

19. Below, record Ms. Begay's BUN and creatinine values at 0800 Sunday from the EPR. What are the implications of these results in regard to target organ damage?

Next, click on **Vital Signs** in the EPR and note the trends in Sally Begay's blood pressure since admission.

20. For each day and time below, record Sally Begay's blood pressure reading.

Day and Time	BP	Day and Time	BP
Saturday 1600		Tuesday 0800	
Saturday 2400		Tuesday 1600	
Sunday 0800		Tuesday 2400	
Sunday 1600		Wednesday 0800	
Sunday 2400		Wednesday 1600	
Monday 0800		Wednesday 2400	
Monday 1600		Thursday 0800	
Monday 2400		Thursday 1600	
		Thursday 2400	

21. What trend is emerging in the above blood pressure readings? How can this be explained?

 22. Consider the medication therapy recommendations of the Joint National Committee on prevention, detection, evaluation and treatment of high blood pressure (discussed on p. 763 in your textbook). Compare recommended protocol with the treatment being used for Sally Begay. Given all you have learned so far, do you think her treatment is consistent with the textbook picture? Explain.

➡ Sally Begay is scheduled for discharge Friday. You will be participating in her discharge teaching, specifically addressing how to manage her hypertension. Close the EPR and open her chart. Click on **Health Team** to read the reports written by the nurse case manager, clinical nurse specialist, and social worker.

23. The following chart outlines lifestyle modifications that may be necessary to control hypertension. Next to each, indicate whether Sally Begay could benefit from teaching in this area. For items checked as "Yes," provide suggestions for discharge teaching.

Lifestyle Modification	Yes	No	Recommended Teaching for Items Checked "Yes"
Weight reduction	____	____	
Sodium restriction	____	____	
Dietary fat reduction	____	____	
Exercise	____	____	
Alcohol restriction	____	____	
Caffeine restriction	____	____	
Relaxation techniques	____	____	
Smoking cessation	____	____	
Potassium supplementation	____	____	

24. You are concerned that Sally Begay may not continue to follow the treatment plan once she returns to her rural home, despite the health team's notes that indicate arrangements have been made for community care follow-up. What additional ideas could you consider in developing a culturally sensitive plan of care upon discharge?

Chronic Arterial Occlusive Disease

👓 **Reading Assignment:** Vascular Problems (Chapter 25)

Patient: Carmen Gonzales, Room 302

In this lesson you will explore chronic arterial occlusive disease as it relates to Carmen Gonzales, a 56-year-old Hispanic female patient who has type 2 diabetes mellitus (DM). Because DM can accelerate the process of atherosclerosis, she is at increased risk for chronic arterial occlusive disease. It will be helpful to have a drug reference book available for use during this lesson.

✏️ **Writing Activity**

1. How does atherosclerotic plaque lead to chronic arterial occlusive disease?

2. Identify and describe the classic symptom of chronic arterial occlusive disease.

3. What are other symptoms of chronic arterial occlusive disease?

CD-ROM Activity

Go to the Supervisor's Office and sign in to work with Carmen Gonzales on Tuesday at 0700. Next proceed to the Nurses' Station and find the location of report by clicking on the bulletin board. Go to that location and listen to the report on Carmen Gonzales, recording any information pertaining to arterial disease below.

Student Notes

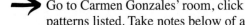 Return to the Nurses' Station and open Ms. Gonzales' chart. Click on **History and Physical** and read the entire report.

4. Based on the data gathered from report and from the History and Physical, what risk factors does Carmen Gonzales have for chronic arterial occlusive disease? Which of these risk factors can be controlled or modified?

Go to Carmen Gonzales' room, click on **Health History**, and obtain data in each of the health patterns listed. Take notes below of any data that relate to arterial disease.

Student Notes

Now click on **Physical** and complete a physical examination of the patient's abdomen and lower extremities.

> 5. Use the space below to record the data you obtain during Carmen Gonzales' physical examination. Then chart your findings in the EPR.

Abdomen and Lower Extremities	Tuesday 0700 Data

Bowel sounds

Palpation

Edema

Dorsalis pedis pulse

Posterior-tibial pulse

Skin check

> 6. Carmen Gonzales obviously had the left leg wound at home for several days before admission. Why is it important to determine how she treated the leg wound before she came to the hospital?

 7. What diagnostic tests would be useful to evaluate Carmen Gonzales' chronic arterial occlusive disease? *Hint:* See p. 772 in the textbook.

➡ Return to Carmen Gonzales' chart and click on **Physicians' Orders**. Read the admission orders written on Sunday.

8. What medication did the physician specifically order to treat her leg infection?

9. To what extent does the ordered medication dose and time correlate with the recommendations found in a drug reference book? Briefly explain your answer.

10. What four other classes of pharmacologic agents could Carmen Gonzales' physician order to treat her chronic arterial occlusive disease? Give at least one example for each medication class. *Hint:* Refer to Table 25-6 on p. 773 of the textbook if needed.

11. It is time to develop a plan of nursing care for Carmen Gonzales. Using all of the data you have gathered, write three nursing diagnostic statements and associated goals/outcomes and nursing interventions. Record these below and on the next page.

Nursing Diagnosis #1 _____ **related to** _____

Goals/Outcomes

Nursing Interventions

Nursing Diagnosis #2 _____ **related to** _____

Goals/Outcomes

Nursing Interventions

Nursing Diagnosis #3 _____ **related to** _____

Goals/Outcomes

Nursing Interventions

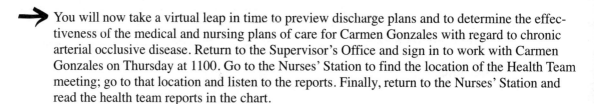

You will now take a virtual leap in time to preview discharge plans and to determine the effectiveness of the medical and nursing plans of care for Carmen Gonzales with regard to chronic arterial occlusive disease. Return to the Supervisor's Office and sign in to work with Carmen Gonzales on Thursday at 1100. Go to the Nurses' Station to find the location of the Health Team meeting; go to that location and listen to the reports. Finally, return to the Nurses' Station and read the health team reports in the chart.

12. What data in the health team reports specifically address Ms. Gonzales' chronic arterial occlusive disease? Explain possible reasons for the amount of detail you heard.

To determine how well the infection has been controlled in Carmen Gonzales' arterial leg ulcer, access the EPR and evaluate her vital signs and pain level since Sunday at 2400.

13. Below, record the vital signs and blood glucose levels charted in the EPR at the specified dates and times. Record NR for any data that were not recorded.

	Sunday 2400	Monday 2000	Tuesday 2000	Wednesday 2000
Temperature (F)				
Heart rate				
Blood pressure				
Respiratory rate				
Oxygen saturation				
Oxygen source				
Pain rating, source, and characteristics				
Blood glucose				

14. Based on the data you recorded in question 13, what interventions have been successful to this point in controlling Carmen Gonzales' infection in her left lower leg ulcer? What data support your answer? What areas of her care warrant continued attention?

LESSON **20**

Diabetes Mellitus Part 1

👓 **Reading Assignment:** Assessment of the Endocrine System (Chapter 28)
Diabetes Mellitus and Hypoglycemia (Chapter 30)

Patient: Carmen Gonzales, Room 302

In this lesson you have been assigned to care for Carmen Gonzales, a 56-year-old Hispanic female patient who was admitted to the hospital because of an infected left lower leg and type 2 diabetes mellitus (DM). Have a drug handbook ready to use as a supplemental reference as you complete this lesson.

📖 Before you begin, review general introductory information about DM in your textbook. Then answer the following questions.

1. Describe DM and the basis for the resulting abnormalities in carbohydrate, protein, and fat metabolism.

2. Briefly define and summarize the pathophysiologic differences between type 1 and type 2 DM.

Type 1 DM

Type 2 DM

3. Highlight the distinguishing features of type 1 and type 2 DM by completing the chart below and on the next page. *Hint:* Refer to textbook Table 30-2 for help if needed.

Features	Type 1 DM	Type 2 DM
Insulin status		
Age		
Clinical presentation		
Body build		
Family history		
Islet cell antibodies		
Human leukocyte antigen (HLA) association		
Incidence		
Symptoms		
Ketones		

Features	Type 1 DM	Type 2 DM
Complications		
Treatment		
Racial distribution		

CD-ROM Activity

In the Supervisor's Office, sign in to work with Ms. Gonzales on Tuesday at 0700. Go to the Nurses' Station, open her chart, and click on **History and Physical**. Read the entire report, including the Emergency Department Record. (Remember to scroll down to read all pages.)

4. What data in the chart specifically address Carmen Gonzales and her DM?

5. What other information specific to DM would you have gathered if you had been present during the ED assessment?

6. As listed below and on the next page, Carmen Gonzales has coronary artery disease, hypertension, and congestive heart failure; she also had a severe right leg infection within the past 5 months. Indicate whether or not each problem directly relates to her diabetes. Briefly explain each answer.

Problem	Relates to DM? (Yes or No)	Rationale for Answer
CAD		
Hypertension		

Problem	Relates to DM? (Yes or No)	Rationale for Answer
CHF		
R leg infection		

7. Is Carmen Gonzales in a racial group that is at high risk for DM? Briefly explain your answer. *Hint:* Refer to Table 30-4 on p. 932 in the textbook if needed.

8. Below are clinical manifestations of DM identified in the textbook. In column 2, indicate (with Yes or No) whether each manifestation is usually present in type 2 DM. Then indicate (with Yes or No) whether Carmen Gonzales displays each manifestation. (Return to her chart for help if needed.)

Clinical Manifestation	Present in Type 2 DM? (Yes or No)	Experienced by Carmen Gonzales? (Yes or No)
Polyuria		
Polydipsia		
Polyphagia		
Visual blurring		
Fatigue		
Weight loss		
Coma		
Chronic complications		

9. To what degree does Carmen Gonzales fit the typical clinical picture of a patient with type 2 diabetes mellitus?

10. What two tests could be used to determine Carmen Gonzales' control of DM? What is the purpose for each of the tests? How often should they be done? *Hint:* See textbook pp. 937–938 if needed.

Click on **Physicians' Orders** in Carmen Gonzales' chart and review the orders.

11. Identify those written orders that relate specifically to managing her diabetes.

Next, click on **Expired MARs** and review the medications charted there.

12. How many times and in what doses was insulin given to Carmen Gonzales?

13. If Carmen Gonzales does not take insulin at home, why has it been ordered for her during this hospitalization? What has changed?

14. As part of clinical preparation, read about glyburide and regular insulin in your drug reference book. Then fill in the missing pieces of information in the following drug cards.

Drug Card

Generic Name: Glyburide

Trade Names:

Mechanism of Action:

Dosage:

Routes of Administration:

Key Patient Teaching Points:

Drug Card

Generic Name: Regular insulin

Trade Names:

Mechanism of Action:

Dosage:

Routes of Administration:

Key Patient Teaching Points:

→ Close Carmen Gonzales' chart and open her MAR.

15. Determine which routine medications you will be administering to Carmen Gonzales during the Tuesday 0700 to 1500 shift. List below the medications you must give her, the reason for giving each, and the time each is due. Use your drug handbook if needed.

Medication	Reason for Giving	Time Due

→ The night staff nurse is now ready to give report on Carmen Gonzales. Close the MAR, check the bulletin board to find the location of report, and go to that room to listen to report. Use the space below to take notes from the report about data related to her diabetes.

Student Notes

16. What thoughts do you have about the report you received? Are there additional data about her diabetes mellitus that you think should have been included? If so, what?

→ After report, go to Carmen Gonzales room and click on **Vital Signs**. Take a set of vital signs and return to the Nurses' Station to record them in the EPR.

17. Based on data identified from taking the vital signs, you determine that Carmen Gonzales needs to have which PRN medication administered at this time? Explain your rationale.

→ It is now time to administer 0800 medications to Carmen Gonzales. Go back to her room and click on **Medications** to fulfill this nursing responsibility.

18. What is the rationale for giving the glyburide at 0800? (Refer to your textbook, drug reference book, or the drug card you completed in question 14 if needed.)

19. The shift charge nurse tells you that Carmen Gonzales received 6 units of regular insulin SC for a blood glucose level of 260 mg/dl while you were listening to report. Investigate the information below regarding regular insulin in your drug handbook or textbook, and fill in the chart so it will be available to refer if needed during your shift.

	Expected Length of Time	**Actual Time after 0730 Dose**
Onset		
Peak		
Duration		

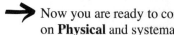 Now you are ready to complete a physical examination of Carmen Gonzales. In her room, click on **Physical** and systematically assess each of the areas by clicking on **Head and Neck**, **Chest/Upper Extremities**, and **Abdomen and Lower Extremities**.

20. Record the results of your physical examination below. Then go to the Nurses' Station and access Carmen Gonzales' EPR. Click on **Assessments**, and enter your physical examination findings in the box in the lower right screen, using the key code in the box on the right.

Assessment Area	Findings

Head and Neck

Chest/Upper Extremities

Abdomen and Lower Extremities

21. Do any of your findings in question 20 deviate from what you expected? Explain.

Diabetes Mellitus
Part 2

👓 **Reading Assignment:** Assessment of the Endocrine System (Chapter 28)
Diabetes Mellitus and Hypoglycemia (Chapter 30)

Patient: Carmen Gonzales, Room 302

In this lesson you will continue to care for Carmen Gonzales, a 56-year-old female with type 2 diabetes mellitus (DM) who was admitted for an infected leg that became gangrenous. If you have not done so already, please complete Lesson 20 before beginning this one. Have a drug handbook ready to use as a reference during this lesson.

💿 **CD-ROM Activity**

Go to the Supervisor's Office and sign in to work again with Carmen Gonzales, this time for the Thursday 0700 shift. Next, go to the Nurses' Station and open her chart to update yourself about her care since you were last assigned to her on Tuesday. Specifically, click on the following areas as part of your review: **Physicians' Orders**, **Physicians' Notes**, **Nurses' Notes**, and **Expired MARs**. When you have finished your review, close the chart and access the MAR in the blue notebook. Determine which regularly scheduled medications you will give to Carmen Gonzales today during the 0700 to 1500 shift.

1. In the area below, identify the routine medications you will be giving today, the time the dose is due, and why you will be giving it.

Medication Order	Time Due	Why It Is Being Given

2. When did the physician order furosemide (Lasix) for Carmen Gonzales? What was the rationale for the order and what effect might it have on her DM? (Use your drug handbook if needed to answer this question).

→ The night nurse is ready to give report on Carmen Gonzales. Check the bulletin board for the location of report for this patient and go there to hear the report. Listen for information that relates to her diabetes as well as to her general condition.

3. How satisfied were you with the report you heard? Is there anything you wish the night nurse would have included about Ms. Gonzales' DM? If so, what?

4. It is now time to obtain vital signs on Carmen Gonzales. Go to her room to measure 0800 vital signs and record them in the area below and also on the EPR. Compare these values with previous readings to determine her stability.

Blood pressure _____   Heart rate _____   Oxygen saturation _____

Temperature _____   Respiratory rate _____   Pain rating _____

→ Return to Carmen Gonzales' room and administer her 0800 medications. The registered nurse who is also assigned to the care of Carmen Gonzales has invited you to participate in the patient's discharge planning. You accept at once, indicating that you will first need to collect more data. In the patient's room, click on **Health History** to conduct the patient interview. As you conduct your assessment, focus particularly on data that will be helpful in planning for discharge needs related to DM.

5. Record (below and on the next two pages) the data you collect from the health history that will help you develop a plan of care for Carmen Gonzales.

Health History Section	**Patient Data**
Perception/Self-Concept	

Health History Section	Patient Data

Activity

Sexuality/Reproduction

Culture

Nutrition-Metabolic

Sleep-Rest

Health History Section	Patient Data
Role/Relationship	
Health Perception	
Elimination	
Cognitive/Perceptual	
Coping/Stress	
Value/Belief	

6. Now that you have considered the information gathered over time from Carmen Gonzales' medical history, health history interview, and physical examinations, how will these data influence the way you proceed with your discharge teaching in relation to DM? Refer back to the patient's chart and EPR as needed.

7. How do the culture-specific data you gathered influence your discharge teaching?

8. Below and on the next page, develop two nursing diagnoses for Carmen Gonzales that relate to diabetes and its self-management. Write goals and sample interventions for each nursing diagnosis. *Hint:* Use the Nursing Care Plan: Patient with Diabetes Mellitus (textbook pp. 954–957) and adapt it as needed to meet Carmen Gonzales' needs.

Nursing Diagnosis # 1

Goals

Interventions

Nursing Diagnosis # 2

Goals

Interventions

➤ Check the bulletin board in the Nurses' Station for the location of the discharge planning meeting scheduled today for Carmen Gonzales. Attend the meeting and, as a follow-up, read the health team reports in Ms. Gonzales' chart. Focus on information that relates to her needs to manage diabetes at home following discharge.

9. What are Carmen Gonzales' needs with respect to dietary management?

 10. Carmen Gonzales needs to learn how to manage her DM during times of illness. List below and on the next page five teaching points to include in sick-day guidelines. *Hint:* Refer to textbook p. 959.

   a.

   b.

c.

d.

e.

11. To help Carmen Gonzales reduce her risk for developing foot infection because of diabetes mellitus, create a list of actions she should take, using the general categories listed below and on the next page. *Hint:* Use the Patient Teaching Guide on p. 968 in your textbook if needed.

Inspection

Foot care

Foot wear

Measures to avoid injury

Measures to increase general circulation

What to do if you develop a foot problem

12. What information should you provide to Carmen Gonzales to help her reduce her risk for developing the chronic microvascular complications of diabetes mellitus listed below?

Microvascular Complication	What It Is	How to Prevent It
Diabetic retinopathy		
Nephropathy		
Neuropathy		

LESSON **22** ────────────────

Assessment of the Nervous System

────────────────

 Reading Assignment: Assessment of the Nervous System (Chapter 41)

Patients: David Ruskin, Room 303
Andrea Wang, Room 310

In this lesson you will explore the process of neurologic assessment for two patients who have suffered trauma to the neurologic system: David Ruskin, a 32-year-old African-American man who suffered head injury after being struck by an automobile while bicycling, and Andrea Wang, a 20-year-old Asian-American woman who suffered spinal cord injury in a diving accident.

Writing Activity

1. What are five important items to include when taking a patient history as part of a neurologic assessment?

    a.

    b.

    c.

    d.

    e.

2. Identify at least five illnesses to include when asking about family history of neurologic diseases or diseases affecting neurologic status.

    a.

    b.

c.

d.

e.

3. Listed below are four classic neurologic symptoms that should be inquired about during a neurologic health history. For each symptom, identify what to explore during the assessment.

Health History	Items to Include in Assessment
Headache	
Dizziness and vertigo	
Weakness and paresthesia	
Pain	

 4. When you are taking a medication history, which types of medications should be included? Are there specific categories of drugs that should be included in this list? *Hint:* See textbook p. 1302 and refer to a pharmacology reference if needed.

CD-ROM Activity

Go to the Supervisor's Office and sign in to work with David Ruskin on Tuesday at 1100. Next, go to the Nurses' Station and open his chart. Click on **History and Physical** and read the Emergency Department Report.

5. What was David Ruskin's neurologic status upon arrival in the emergency department (ED)?

6. Based on David Ruskin's neurologic data documented in the ED, what equipment was probably used to conduct this examination? *Hint:* Refer to Box 41-1 on p. 1303 in the textbook if needed.

➡ 7. Below, record the data documented in the ED report for the following areas of the initial examination.

Patient history related to chief complaint

Vital signs

Level of consciousness

Pupillary response

Brain stem function (corneal reflex)

Motor and sensory function in all four extremities

8. Why are vital signs important to monitor in a patient with a neurologic problem?

Now click on **Physicians' Orders** and note the diagnostic tests that were ordered to evaluate David Ruskin's head injury.

    9. Two diagnostic tests were ordered for David Ruskin while he was in the ED. What are the differences between these two tests and why were they ordered?

Test	Description and Purpose
Skull series	
CT scan of head	

    10. For each of these diagnostic tests, what precautions should be taken postprocedure?

 Click on **Diagnostics** and read the results of the two studies.

    11. What did the results of the skull series and the CT scan show?

    12. What is a potential problem associated with the use of a CT scan for a patient who has an altered level of consciousness (e.g., is not fully oriented)?

➤ Return to the Supervisor's Office and sign in to work with Andrea Wang on Tuesday at 1100. Go to the Nurses' Station and open her chart. Click on **History and Physical** and read the Emergency Department Report for Sunday at 1230.

13. a. What were Andrea Wang's vital signs on admission?

   Blood pressure _____   Heart rate _____   Oxygen saturation _____

   Temperature _____   Respiratory rate _____

   b. What reason can you give for the alteration noted in her admission vital signs?

14. What data were recorded in the Emergency Department Report for the following areas of the initial examination?

Client history related to chief complaint

Vital signs

Level of consciousness

Pupillary response

Brain stem function (corneal reflex)

Motor and sensory function in all four extremities

15. What data in the Emergency Department Report indicate that Andrea Wang has loss of bowel or bladder function related to her spinal cord injury?

16. What is an MRI? Why was this ordered for Andrea Wang in the emergency department? What were the results?

LESSON 23

Traumatic Brain Injury

⟋ᗺ **Reading Assignment:** Traumatic and Neoplastic Problems of the Brain (Chapter 42)

Patient: David Ruskin, Room 303

In this lesson you are assigned to the care of David Ruskin, a 32-year-old African-American man who suffered a closed head injury, fractured humerus, and scalp lacerations after being struck by an automobile while bicycling. If you have not already completed Lesson 22 on neurologic assessment, you should do so before beginning this lesson.

1. What are the four variables that directly influence the extent of traumatic brain injury (or craniocerebral trauma) sustained by a patient?

   a.

   b.

   c.

   d.

🖸 CD-ROM Activity

Go to the Supervisor's Office and sign in to work with David Ruskin on Tuesday at 0700. Next, go to the Nurse's Station, open his chart, and click on **History and Physical** to read the Emergency Department Report.

2. What is the description of David Ruskin's head injury in the chart? What other data are important to note with regard to the accident and the events that immediately followed?

3. To what extent does David Ruskin fit the profile of the typical patient admitted to the ED with traumatic brain injury? *Hint:* Refer to the discussion under Epidemiology for cranio-cerebral trauma on textbook p. 1351.

4. Review the mechanisms of traumatic brain injury shown below from Fig. 42-12 of the textbook. Circle the picture that represents the type of injury experienced by David Ruskin. Beneath the figure, write the name of that type of injury and briefly describe why it applies to David Ruskin.

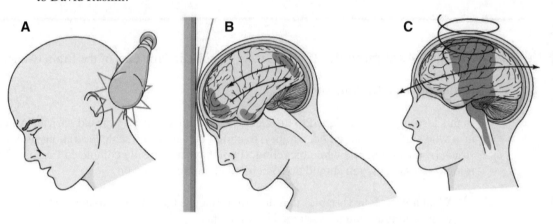

5. Provide a description of David Ruskin's neurologic status during assessment, based on the Emergency Department Report.

6. The following six terms are often used to describe level of consciousness. Circle the term that best fits David Ruskin's level of consciousness and briefly explain your choice. *Hint:* Refer to Box 42-1 on textbook p. 1318 if needed.

Alert   Confused   Lethargic

Obtunded   Stuporous   Comatose

7. What is the Glasgow Coma Scale? What are its three categories, and how is it scored?

8. What were David Ruskin's Glasgow Coma Scale scores in the ED? What interpretation can you make about his neurologic status based on these scores?

9. What is increased intracranial pressure (ICP)? What normally contributes to intracranial pressure in the brain?

Writing Activity

10. Summarize the pathophysiology of increased ICP. *Hint:* Refer to pp. 1329–1332 of your textbook.

11. What are the early and late clinical manifestations of increased ICP? *Hint:* Refer to p. 1332 in your textbook.

12. Why was a CT scan ordered of David Ruskin's head? What were the results?

13. What were David Ruskin's vital signs upon admission?

    Temperature _____   Heart rate _____   Respiratory rate _____

    Blood pressure _____   Oxygen saturation _____

14. What changes would you assess for in David Ruskin's vital signs to alert you that his ICP is increased?

15. If clinical manifestations were severe enough, what medications would you anticipate being ordered to treat increased ICP? What medications should be used cautiously? Briefly explain your answers. *Hint:* Refer to p. 1332 in the textbook if needed.

16. If needed, orders for what two other treatments might be written to help prevent complications related to increased ICP? Briefly explain how they would help.

    a.

    b.

→ Click on **Physicians' Orders** and review the orders that were written for David Ruskin.

17. List the orders that pertain to David Ruskin's diagnosis of closed head injury.

→ Next, click on **Nurses' Notes**. Read the notes written for Sunday and Monday.

18. What documentation did you find in the nurses' notes related to neurologic status?

→ Close the chart and check the bulletin board to see where report will be given for David Ruskin. Go to that location to hear report. Answer questions 19 and 20 based on what you hear.

19. What information was reported that pertained to David Ruskin's neurologic status?

20. Was there anything stated during report that was confusing? Is there other information you would have been interested in hearing about during report? If so, what?

→ Now go to David Ruskin's room to do an assessment of your own. Click on **Vital Signs**, obtain a set of vital sign readings, and record them below.

21. What were David Ruskin's vital signs at 0800?

Blood pressure _____   Heart rate _____   Oxygen saturation _____

Temperature _____   Respiratory rate _____   Pain rating _____

Now click on **Health History**, and then **Cognitive/Perceptual**, and assess the three areas that are part of this pattern. You may take notes about his responses below. (You will use this information to formulate an answer to question 22.) Then return to David Ruskin's chart and review the History and Physical again, noting any data related to neurologic function. Finally, return to the patient's room, click on **Physical**, and conduct a physical examination of David Ruskin, noting any findings that relate to his neurologic status.

Student Notes

22. Based on your review of data from the patient's chart and your room visits, record neurologic findings for David Ruskin in each of the following categories.

Mental status

Pupil size/response

Glasgow Coma Scale

Motor strength

Other cranial nerves assessed

23. You note that it is approximately 36 hours since the time of David Ruskin's injury. Using your assessment findings as a guide, indicate whether you think each of the following types of head injury is likely or unlikely in David Ruskin's case. *Hint:* Refer to the section entitled Secondary Injury on p. 1353 in the textbook for help.

Epidural hematoma

Acute subdural hematoma

Subacute subdural hematoma

24. If you answered "Likely" to any of the choices in question 23, why do you think this type of injury is still possible? What instructions pertaining to the assessment of this injury should be given to the family at discharge? *Hint:* Refer to Patient Teaching: Monitoring the Patient with a Minor Head Injury on textbook p. 1356 if needed.

Spinal Cord Injury
Part 1

👓 **Reading Assignment:** Spinal Cord and Peripheral Nerve Problems (Chapter 44)

Patient: Andrea Wang, Room 310

In this lesson you will explore the emergency management and plan of nursing care for Andrea Wang, a 20-year-old Asian-American woman who suffered spinal cord injury in a diving accident. This lesson simulates the clinical preparation that you might do if you were assigned to the care of this patient. If you have not completed Lesson 22, do so before beginning this lesson. It may be also helpful to have a drug reference book available during the lesson.

💿 **CD-ROM Activity**

Go to the Supervisor's Office and sign in to work with Andrea Wang on Tuesday at 0700. Next, go to the Nurses' Station and open her chart. Click on **History and Physical** and read the entire report, including the Emergency Department Record.

1. According to the ED documentation, what was Andrea Wang's mechanism of injury?

2. For each assessment area below and on the next page, record the neurologic findings recorded in Andrea Wang's chart.

Assessment Area	Neurologic Findings
Pupils	
Glasgow Coma Scale score	
Orientation	

Assessment Area	Neurologic Findings

Cranial nerves

Peripheral nerves

3. What diagnostic studies were done in the ED? What did the results of these tests reveal?

 Review the discussion on spinal cord injury under Etiology on pp. 1404–1408 of the textbook. Then answer the following questions.

4. What type of spinal injury did Andrea Wang experience? Circle the diagram below that illustrates her injury.

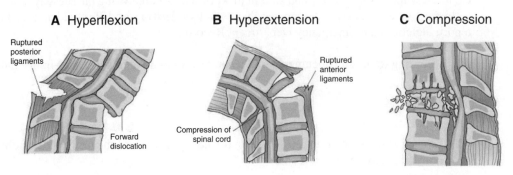

A Hyperflexion   **B** Hyperextension   **C** Compression

Ruptured posterior ligaments

Forward dislocation

Ruptured anterior ligaments

Compression of spinal cord

 Writing Activity

5. Write a brief description of the type of injury you chose in question 4. *Hint:* Refer to p. 1405 of your textbook if needed.

6. Summarize the pathophysiology of spinal cord injury as it affects tissue of the spinal cord. *Hint:* Refer to pp. 1408–1409.

7. What is the level of neurologic injury experienced by Andrea Wang? What functional limitations and sensory impairments will she experience as a result of this injury? *Hint:* Use Figure 44-9 on p. 1410 in your textbook to obtain this information.

8. What type of changes in reflexes should you expect Andrea Wang to exhibit immediately following spinal trauma? What changes are expected as cord edema subsides? What intervention was done in the ED that is associated with loss of function? *Hint:* Refer to p. 1409 of the textbook if needed.

9. What are the five types of syndromes associated with incomplete spinal cord injury? Which of these is Andrea Wang experiencing? Provide a brief rationale for your answer.

10. The Emergency Department Report also states that Andrea Wang is exhibiting spinal shock. What is spinal shock?

→ 11. Below, record the vital signs documented by ED personnel at the time of Andrea Wang's admission. Then indicate whether or not each reading is consistent with changes typically seen in spinal shock. Offer a brief rationale for each decision. *Hint:* Use the discussion on Spinal Shock on p. 2051 and the Medical Management section on p. 2054 in the textbook to formulate your answer.

	Andrea Wang's Results	Consistent with Spinal Shock?	Rationale
Temperature			
Heart rate			
Respiratory rate			
Blood pressure			

12. How long should spinal shock last? How can you determine whether it is resolving?

→ Return to the Emergency Department Report and locate the two therapies listed under the Plan section at the bottom of the first page.

13. What are the two therapies listed?

14. What drug is usually ordered for the steroid protocol, and how is it given? *Hint:* Refer to your drug reference book to find this information.

15. What type of effect should this drug have?

16. What is the beneficial effect of early surgery to decompress and fuse the thoracic spine?

→ Click on **Physicians' Orders** in the chart and review the orders written on Monday.

17. Below, transcribe the six orders that do not relate to medications and indicate their purpose.

Orders	Purpose
a.	
b.	
c.	
d.	
e.	
f.	

Close the chart and find the MAR in the blue notebook on the counter. Open the MAR and find the medications listed for Andrea Wang.

18. For each of the medications listed below and on the next page, identify the classification of the medication and explain why Ms. Wang is receiving it. *Hint:* Use your drug reference book for help.

Medication	Classification	Why Ordered
Famotidine		
Docusate sodium		
Bisacodyl suppository		
Multiple vitamin with minerals		
Vitamin C		
Enoxaparin		
Baclofen		

Medication	Classification	Why Ordered
Acetaminophen		
Oxycodone/ acetaminophen		

➤ Close the MAR and return to the chart to investigate nursing data obtained for Andrea Wang since admission. Click on **Nurses' Notes** and read through the notes in this section.

19. What concerns emerge from the documentation you have just read?

20. After analyzing the data that you have gathered so far in this lesson, develop a list of at least six nursing diagnoses for Andrea Wang that focus on some of the problems that are evident immediately following her spinal cord injury and that may apply during SCI rehabilitation. *Hint:* Refer to p. 1417 in the textbook if needed.

    a.

    b.

    c.

    d.

    e.

    f.

Spinal Cord Injury
Part 2

∩○∞ **Reading Assignment:** Spinal Cord and Peripheral Nerve Problems (Chapter 44)

Patient: Andrea Wang, Room 310

In this lesson you will participate in the nursing management of Andrea Wang, a 20-year-old Asian-American woman who suffered spinal cord injury in a diving accident. If you have not already completed Lesson 22 and Lesson 24, do so before beginning this lesson.

🖥 CD-ROM Activity

Go to the Supervisor's Office and sign in to work with Andrea Wang on Tuesday at 0700. Next, go to the Nurses' Station and find the location where report is being given on this patient. Go there and listen to the report. Consider questions 1 and 2 below as you listen.

1. What information was given in report that is pertinent to the care you will deliver to Andrea Wang this morning?

2. Was there information given in report that was inconsistent in any way? What other questions did you have after report that you wish the nurse had addressed? Describe.

→ Go to Andrea Wang's room and click on **Vital Signs**. Measure her vital signs and record the results below. Also, go to the Nurses' Station and record your findings in the EPR.

3. Blood pressure _____   Heart rate _____   Oxygen saturation _____

   Temperature _____   Respiratory rate _____   Pain rating _____

4. Based on the vital signs you just charted, what nursing intervention is appropriate?

→ It is time to perform a physical assessment of Andrea Wang and administer her medications. To best organize your time, access the MAR in the blue notebook in the Nurses' Station and review the medications that are scheduled for your shift. Then return to her room and click on **Physical**. Observe as the nurse examines each of the areas; record your findings in question 5.

5. Record Andrea Wang's physical examination findings on Tuesday morning. Are any of these unexpected or out of the ordinary?

Area Examined	Findings
Head and Neck	
Chest/Upper Extremities	
Abdomen and Lower Extremities	

→ Now click on **Medications** and then on **Administer**.

6. Which routine medication due at 0900 did the nurse fail to administer?

→ Click on **Health History** and conduct a complete interview with Andrea Wang. As you proceed, record your findings in question 7 (below and on the next page).

7. What significant data did you find as you collected the health history?

Health History Section	Patient Data
Perception/Self-Concept	
Activity	
Sexuality/Reproduction	
Culture	
Nutrition-Metabolic	
Sleep-Rest	
Role/Relationship	

Health History Section	Patient Data
Health Perception	
Elimination	
Cognitive/Perceptual	
Coping/Stress	
Value/Belief	

8. Briefly review all the data you have gathered today from the vital signs, the health history, and the physical examination. In the left column below, transcribe the nursing diagnoses that you generated for question 20 at the end of Lesson 24. Based on the conclusions you have drawn from the newly acquired data, write a revised list of nursing diagnoses in the right column below.

Original Nursing Diagnoses	Revised Nursing Diagnoses

➡ To get the most from this lesson, we will now take a virtual leap in time. Return to the Supervisor's Office and sign in to work with Andrea Wang, this time for Thursday at 1100. Then check the bulletin board in the Nurses' Station for the location of intershift report. Go there and listen to report.

9. What significant data were mentioned in the report on Andrea Wang?

➡ Next, click on **Health Team Meeting** and listen to the reports on Andrea Wang. Record relevant data in question 10. Then go to the Nurses' Station, open her chart, and click on **Health Team** to read each member's written report. Record any additional concerns in question 10.

10. What are the primary concerns of the health team members listed below?

Case manager

Social worker

Clinical nurse specialist

11. The clinical nurse specialist and other nurses mention the need to monitor Andrea Wang for autonomic dysreflexia. Briefly explain what this is, how you would recognize it when it occurs, and what you would do to manage it. *Hint:* Refer to pp. 1425–1426 if needed.

Click on **Nurses' Notes** and read the notes from Tuesday until today.

12. What are the current issues involved in Andrea Wang's care?

13. Part of the plan of care for Andrea Wang is to implement a teaching plan about measures to prevent autonomic dysreflexia. What will you include in this discussion?

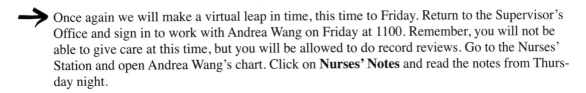 Once again we will make a virtual leap in time, this time to Friday. Return to the Supervisor's Office and sign in to work with Andrea Wang on Friday at 1100. Remember, you will not be able to give care at this time, but you will be allowed to do record reviews. Go to the Nurses' Station and open Andrea Wang's chart. Click on **Nurses' Notes** and read the notes from Thursday night.

14. What complication developed?

15. What was the most likely reason for this occurrence?

 16. What manifestations were present to suggest that this complication was occurring? Were these manifestations consistent with the ones in your textbook? Explain.

LESSON **26**

Musculoskeletal Trauma

 Reading Assignment: Assessment of the Musculoskeletal System (Chapter 45)
Trauma to the Musculoskeletal System (Chapter 46)

Patient: David Ruskin, Room 303

In this lesson you will care for David Ruskin, a 31-year-old patient who was hit by a car while bicycling. He sustained a fractured right humerus during this trauma.

1. The initial clinical manifestations following a fracture are listed below and on the next page. Briefly discuss the basis for each manifestation. *Hint:* Refer to Clinical Manifestations: Fracture on textbook p. 1469 if needed.

Clinical Manifestation	Basis for the Manifestation
Pain	
Loss of normal function	
Obvious deformity	
Excessive motion at site	

Clinical Manifestation	Basis for the Manifestation
Soft tissue edema	
Warmth over injured area	
Ecchymosis	
Impairment or loss of sensation or paralysis	
Shock	

CD-ROM Activity

Go to the Supervisor's Office and sign in to work with David Ruskin on Tuesday at 0700. Next, go to the Nurses' Station and open his chart. Click on **History and Physical** and read the entire report, including the Emergency Department Report. Think about what data found in this report relates to musculoskeletal trauma.

2. In addition to data about manifestations described in the textbook (question 1), what other findings in the Emergency Department Report relate to the fractured humerus?

3. Review the three other injuries (besides the fractured humerus) cited in the Emergency Department Report. Below and on the next page, in order of priority for nursing assessment and management, list all four of the injuries that were identified. Describe how each of the other injuries may affect assessment of the fractured humerus.

   a.

b.

c.

d.

 4. In what stage of bone healing is David Ruskin immediately after hospitalization? What are the factors that could affect healing of his fractured humerus? *Hint:* Refer to textbook p. 1469 and Table 46-1 on p. 1470 if needed.

Click on **Diagnostics** in David Ruskin's chart. Read the Radiological Report for Sunday at 1600.

5. Note the type of fracture that is documented in the AP/lateral right humerus x-ray that was done prior to David Ruskin's surgery. Circle the diagram below that matches the term for the fracture found in the diagnostic report. Write the name of the type of fracture below the diagram.

<table>
<tr><td>**A**</td><td>**B**</td><td>**C**</td></tr>
<tr><td>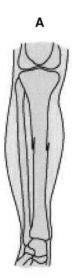</td><td>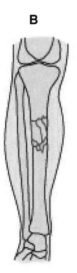</td><td>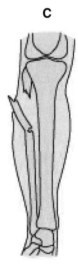</td></tr>
</table>

6. What method of fracture reduction did David Ruskin undergo? What is involved with this type of reduction? *Hint:* Refer to p. 1474 in your textbook.

→ Check the bulletin board in the Nurses' Station to find the location for morning report for David Ruskin. Go to that location and listen to the report.

7. What significant data were presented in morning report? *Hint:* Refer back to Chapter 18 of your textbook or Lesson 11 in this workbook to review postoperative data to monitor.

8. What area(s) of inconsistency did you notice in the report? What information was missing that should have been included?

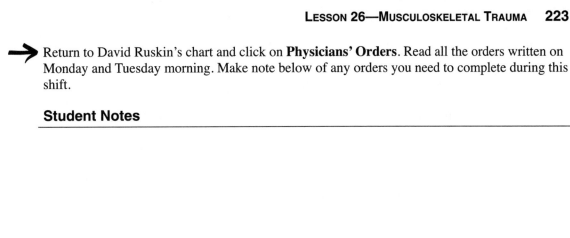

Return to David Ruskin's chart and click on **Physicians' Orders**. Read all the orders written on Monday and Tuesday morning. Make note below of any orders you need to complete during this shift.

Student Notes

9. What is the rationale for the use of the "sky hook" or for keeping the affected arm elevated on a pillow?

10. How will you know that the "sky hook" and the limb elevation with pillow are having their intended effect?

➡ Now go to David Ruskin's room and obtain a full set of vital sign readings.

11. Write the vital signs below and then record them in the EPR.

    Blood pressure _____ Heart rate _____ Oxygen saturation _____

    Temperature _____ Respiratory rate _____ Pain rating _____

➡ Based on the pain rating, you decide that Mr. Ruskin needs to be medicated. Go to the Nurses' Station, open the MAR, and find the medications listed for Mr. Ruskin's pain.

12. Which of the medications listed in the MAR will you administer to David Ruskin, and why?

➡ Go to David Ruskin's room and medicate him for pain. Click on **Medications** and give the appropriate medication. Be sure to wait 30 minutes for the medication to work before doing a physical assessment! Click on **Physical** and perform a complete bedside physical exam.

13. Record your findings from David Ruskin's physical exam in the areas below and on the next page.

Area Examined   **Findings**

Head and Neck

Chest/Upper Extremities

Area Examined	Findings
Abdomen and Lower Extremities	

14. Based on the results of your examination, what interventions are most appropriate at this time? Be sure to address any physician orders that also need attention at this time.

15. Listed below and on the next page are potential complications after fracture. Consider the location of David Ruskin's fracture and circle Yes or No in the second column to indicate whether or not that complication is likely to occur to Mr. Ruskin. Provide your rationale for each answer and a brief description of how each complication would manifest.

Complication of Fracture	High Risk for Occurrence?	Rationale for Answer	How You Would Recognize This Complication?
Nerve injury	Yes No		
Fracture blister	Yes No		

Complication of Fracture	High Risk for Occurrence?	Rationale for Answer	How You Would Recognize This Complication?
Fat embolism syndrome	Yes No		
Compartment syndrome	Yes No		
Impaired fracture healing	Yes No		
Infection	Yes No		
Heterotropic bone formation	Yes No		
Complex regional pain syndrome	Yes No		

➡ Return to the Supervisor's Office and sign in to work with David Ruskin again at Thursday at 1100. Find the location of the health team meeting on Mr. Ruskin. Go to that room and listen to all the reports about his status for discharge (see question 16 below). Then go to the Nurses' Station, open his chart, and click on **Health Team** to read the written reports.

16. Before David Ruskin is discharged to home on Friday, what teaching does he need related to the fractured humerus? Be sure to take into account all you have learned about him thus far. *Hint:* Review the Patient/Family Education section on p. 1483 in the textbook if needed.

➡ Before you proceed with discharge plans, you wish to be certain that David Ruskin's fracture is healing without incident. Open his EPR and click on **Hematology**.

17. What is the WBC count?

18. What is the significance of this finding?

➡ Next, click on **Vital Signs** and note his temperature. Review the trend over the last several days.

19. What conclusion can you draw after analyzing the temperatures?

20. How do the WBC count and temperature trends correlate with the incidence of post-operative complications following open reduction of fracture?

Degenerative Disorders

 Reading Assignment: Assessment of the Musculoskeletal System (Chapter 45)
Degenerative Disorders (Chapter 47)

Patient: Carmen Gonzales, Room 302

In this lesson you will explore the assessment and management of a patient diagnosed with osteomyelitis. You will be working with Carmen Gonzales, who developed osteomyelitis as a consequence of a nonhealing leg ulcer that became gangrenous. It will be helpful to have a drug handbook available as a reference during this lesson.

Before you begin, review the process for assessing musculoskeletal manifestations. Refer to the Assessment section of textbook Chapter 45 (p. 1453) if needed.

1. List 11 items that should be included when conducting a history of the current problem when a patient seeks treatment for a musculoskeletal condition.

   a.

   b.

   c.

   d.

   e.

   f.

   g.

   h.

   i.

   j.

   k.

2. When taking a health history for a patient with a musculoskeletal problem, identify information that is important to elicit in each of the following selected areas.

Nutrition

Occupation

Exercise regimen

Ability to perform ADLs

Physical layout of home

Medications

Match each of the following tests useful in diagnosing musculoskeletal problems with its appropriate description.

3. _____ X-ray

4. _____ Magnetic resonance imaging

5. _____ Arthrography

6. _____ Bone scan

7. _____ Indium imaging

8. _____ Arthrocentesis

9. _____ Arthroscopy

10. _____ Biopsy

a. A radiologic examination of soft tissue joint structures to diagnose trauma to joint capsules or supporting ligaments.

b. A method of aspirating synovial fluid, blood, or pus via a needle inserted into the joint cavity.

c. Skeletal imaging done after injecting the patient with a radioisotope, such as technetium 99.

d. Removal and examination of a sample of tissue to detect disorders such as cancer or infection of the bone.

e. A film taken with either an anteroposterior or lateral view to detect or follow progress of a musculoskeletal problem.

f. Allows endoscopic examination of various joints using a fiberoptic instrument.

g. Involves using a substance that is tagged to leukocytes to detect bone infection.

h. Uses magnetic fields to diagnose many conditions affecting tendons, ligaments, cartilage, and bone marrow.

11. What is osteomyelitis?

 CD-ROM Activity

Go to the Supervisor's Office and sign in to work with Carmen Gonzales on Tuesday at 0700. Next, go to the Nurses' Station and open her chart. Click on **History and Physical**; read the entire report, including the Emergency Department Report. Look for any data related to musculoskeletal function.

12. What clinical manifestations of osteomyelitis does Carmen Gonzales have upon presentation to the ED?

13. How does her documented set of clinical manifestations of osteomyelitis compare with those presented in the textbook chapter? *Hint:* Refer to textbook p. 1569 if needed.

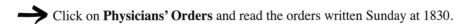 Click on **Physicians' Orders** and read the orders written Sunday at 1830.

14. Identify three diagnostic and/or laboratory tests that were ordered related to the diagnosis of osteomyelitis, and identify any particular postprocedure care that should be done following these tests. *Hint:* If you need to recall concepts regarding inflammation and infection, refer back to Chapter 11 of the textbook and/or Lesson 5 of this workbook.

15. What surgical procedure is ordered that is most likely related (directly or indirectly) to this diagnosis?

 Click on **Diagnostics** and review the Radiological Report for Sunday at 1600.

 16. What documentation on the Radiological Report relates to the diagnosis of osteomyelitis? What is your interpretation of this finding? (*Hint:* Synthesize information you read in textbook Chapters 45 and 47 to develop your answer).

    a. Documented report

    b. Interpretation of this finding

 Click on **Surgeon's Notes** and read the entire report for Monday at 1330.

 17. The textbook includes surgery as a treatment modality during the discussion on osteomyelitis on p. 1570. What is the purpose of surgical intervention in osteomyelitis? Did Ms. Gonzales' surgery involve debridement of bone or of soft tissue only? How do you think this surgical procedure will assist her to recover from osteomyelitis?

➜ Close the chart and click on the bulletin board to find the location of the morning intershift report for Carmen Gonzales. Go to that location and listen to the report.

18. Record any significant information from report in the space below. This data will be broad-based in that it will consider Ms. Gonzales' pertinent history as well as postoperative data that should be monitored. *Hint:* Refer back to Chapter 18 of your textbook or Lesson 8 in this workbook if you need to review postoperative data important to monitor.

19. What other information related to osteomyelitis do you wish the nurse had included in the intershift report, if any?

➜ Go to Carmen Gonzales' room, click on **Vital Signs**, and obtain a full set of vital signs.

20. Record the vital signs readings you obtained below. Also record these findings in the EPR.

Temperature _____   Heart rate _____   Blood pressure _____

Respiratory rate _____   Oxygen saturation _____   Pain rating _____

➜ Go to the Nurses' Station and access Carmen Gonzales' MAR. Read the medication orders for Tuesday.

21. Which of the medications should be given to Ms. Gonzales based on her vital signs results in question 20? Explain your rationale.

22. Note that Carmen Gonzales is also scheduled to receive cefoxitin at 0800 and that she has an IV infusion running. The premixed bag of IV medication is labeled "Cefoxitin 2 grams in 50 mL of 5% dextrose in water."

   a. What type of medication is this, and why is it ordered for this patient?

   b. Is this solution compatible with the solution ordered in the primary IV line? (*Hint:* Refer to your drug handbook at this time if needed.)

   c. Over what amount of time should you infuse this medication?

   d. Your healthcare agency uses IV infusion pumps for all IV medications given by IV piggyback. At how many mL per hour should you set the pump to deliver the medication at a safe infusion rate?

➤ You are interested in how effective the cefoxitin has been to date in treating Carmen Gonzales' osteomyelitis and debrided leg wound. Open the EPR and note her temperature. Compare the temperature you recorded this morning (question 20) with her temperature as documented on Sunday at 2400.

23. How much of a difference is there between the two temperatures, and what is the significance of this change?

→ Click on **Hematology** in the EPR. Note the WBC counts for Sunday at 2000 and Tuesday at 0800.

24. Identify the direction of the change in the WBC count and interpret the significance of the change.

→ It is now Thursday and you are doing clinical make-up. Go to the Supervisor's Office and sign in to work with Carmen Gonzales at 1100. Next, go to the Nurses' Station and find the location of the health team meeting by clicking on the bulletin board. Read the questions below; then go to the health team meeting and listen to the report given by each member. Return to the Nurses' Station and open Carmen Gonzales' chart. Click on **Health Team** and read the written reports.

25. Focusing on follow-up care for osteomyelitis, what should Ms. Gonzales expect regarding continued antibiotic therapy? *Hint:* Refer to textbook p. 1570 if needed.

26. What types of follow-up diagnostic tests should be anticipated for Ms. Gonzales to determine how well the osteomyelitis is responding to therapy? What changes will occur in these diagnostic test results if therapy is effective?

27. What type of wound care should be anticipated, and what resources might be needed in order to ensure that this occurs following discharge? *Hint:* Review Chapter 62 in your textbook if needed.

28. What are possible consequences of inadequate post-discharge care of osteomyelitis?

Part X—Immunologic Problems

LESSON **28** ——————————————————

Acquired Immunodeficiency Syndrome, Part 1

 Reading Assignment: HIV Infection and AIDS (Chapter 50)

Patient: Ira Bradley, Room 309

In this lesson you are assigned to Ira Bradley, a 43-year-old Caucasian male diagnosed with AIDS, dehydration, *Pneumocystis carinii* pneumonia, candidiasis, and Kaposi's sarcoma. You will explore the diagnosis of AIDS and its manifestations and design a plan of care for Mr. Bradley. This lesson simulates the clinical preparation you would need to provide care to this patient. You should have a drug reference book available to use during this lesson.

✎ **Writing Activity**

1. How does the textbook discriminate between HIV infection and AIDS?

 2. What are the three major modes of transmission for the HIV virus that are identified in the textbook? *Hint:* Refer to p. 1654 if needed.

CD-ROM Activity

Go to the Supervisor's Office and sign in to work with Ira Bradley on Tuesday at 0700. Next, go to the Nurses' Station and open his chart. Click on **History and Physical**, and read the entire report, including the Emergency Department Report.

3. What is the route of transmission by which Ira Bradley contracted the HIV virus, according to the chart?

 4. To what degree does his gender and race fit the demographics for HIV as described in the Epidemiology section in your textbook?

5. To what degree does his route of transmission fit the general description in your textbook?

6. How many years ago did Ira Bradley contract the HIV virus? What was the primary reason for his trip to the ED on Sunday?

7. What four conditions does Ira Bradley have that clearly indicate that he has AIDS rather than positive HIV status? *Hint:* These conditions are listed in textbook Box 50-2: CDC Surveillance Case Definition for AIDS.

8. What laboratory tests are used to diagnose HIV infection? In which order are they done? Once it is known that a person is infected with HIV, what laboratory tests will help track the status of the patient's immune system?

→ Next, click on **Physicians' Orders** and review the initial admission orders for Ira Bradley.

9. According to the Emergency Department Report, the physician identified three opportunistic infections or diseases. For each of these conditions (listed below and on the next page), compare and contrast the manifestations, diagnostics, and treatments provided in your textbook. Then compare this information with what you have learned about Ira Bradley's case through his chart data. *Hint:* Use the information found in *AIDS-Related Opportunistic Infections,* beginning on p. 1673 of your textbook.

Oral Candidiasis	Textbook Data	Ira Bradley's Data
Clinical manifestations		
Diagnostic tests		
Medication therapy		

Pneumocystis Carinii Pneumonia	Textbook Data	Ira Bradley's Data
Clinical manifestations		
Diagnostic tests		
Medication therapy		

Kaposi's Sarcoma	Textbook Data	Ira Bradley's Data
Clinical manifestations		
Diagnostic tests		
Medication therapy		

Medication therapy is an important part of the therapeutic management of a patient with AIDS. Close Ira Bradley's chart and open the MAR in the blue notebook. Find Mr. Bradley's MAR and note the medications ordered for him on Tuesday.

10. For each of the medications ordered for Ira Bradley, determine the classification and the purpose for giving it to him. You will need to consider all the information you have gathered so far in this lesson. *Hint:* Use a drug reference book and Table 50-1 on pp. 1660–1661 in your textbook for assistance.

Medication Order	Classification	Purpose for Ira Bradley
D_5 0.45 NS @ 125 cc/hour		
Zidovudine 1 mg/kg (60 mg) IVPB over 1h, q4h x 24 doses		
Trimethoprim 5 mg/kg (300 mg) and sulfamethoxazole 25 mg/kg (1.5) g IVPB q6h x 16 doses		
Delavirdine myselate 400 mg PO TID		
Saquinovir 1200 mg PO TID within 2h of eating		
Fluconazole 100 mg PO in AM x 14 days		
Hydroxyurea 1500 mg PO QD		
Alitretinoin gel 0.1%, apply to lesions BID		

At this time you need to gather nursing assessment data to organize a plan of care for Ira Bradley. Close the MAR and access the EPR. Click on **Admissions** and review the Admissions Profile for Ira Bradley. Use the space below to record any notes about data related to AIDS that will be helpful in developing nursing diagnoses and a plan of nursing care.

Student Notes

11. It is now time to develop a plan of nursing care for Ira Bradley. Your textbook highlights seven nursing diagnoses that commonly apply to a patient who has AIDS. They are listed below and on the next page. Place a check mark next to each one that applies to Ira Bradley. For each diagnosis you choose, complete the nursing diagnostic statement and suggest outcome statements and interventions for his care.

Nursing Diagnosis	Goals/Outcomes	Interventions
Risk for Impaired Gas Exchange related to		
Risk for Infection: Opportunistic (in addition to candida) related to		

Nursing Diagnosis	Goals/Outcomes	Interventions
Imbalanced Nutrition: Less Than Body Requirements related to		
Risk for Deficient Fluid Volume related to		
Activity Intolerance related to		
Anxiety related to		
Risk for Impaired Skin Integrity related to		

Acquired Immunodeficiency Syndrome, Part 2

⌒○⌒ **Reading Assignment:** HIV Infection and AIDS (Chapter 50)

Patient: Ira Bradley, Room 309

In this lesson you will continue to care for Ira Bradley, a 43-year-old Caucasian male diagnosed with acquired immunodeficiency syndrome (AIDS), dehydration, *Pneumocystis carinii* pneumonia, candidiasis, and Kaposi's sarcoma. If you have not done so already, please first complete Lesson 28, which guides you to develop a plan of care for Mr. Bradley. In this lesson, you will focus on assisting in his care.

CD-ROM Activity

Go to the Supervisor's Office and sign in to work with Ira Bradley on Tuesday at 0700. Next, go to the Nurses' Station and check the bulletin board to find the location where report will be given for Ira Bradley. Go to that location and listen to the report. Below, make note of data related to his health problems that will be pertinent to your care.

Student Notes

---

1. Analyze the notes you wrote on the previous page. Is there any information missing that should have been included? Was there any information that was not helpful to you? Explain.

→ It is now 0720. Go to the Nurses' Station and open the MAR in the blue notebook on the counter. Find Ira Bradley's ordered medications.

2. For each of the regularly scheduled medications listed below, identify the time(s) that the medication is due on this shift. For any PRN medications, calculate the earliest time that they can be given, taking into account the time of the last charted dose.

Medication Order	Time(s) Due on This Shift
Zidovudine 60 mg IVPB over 1h q4h X 24 doses	
Trimethoprim 300 mg + sulfamethoxazole 1500 mg IVPB q6h X 16 doses	
Delavirdine myselate 400 mg PO TID	
Saquinovir 1200 mg PO TID within 2h of eating	
Fluconazole 100 mg PO in AM X 14 days	
Hydroxyurea 1500 mg PO QD	
Alitretinoin gel 0.1% apply to lesions BID	
PRN medications	

→ You decide to take 0800 vital signs while the coassigned RN gives 0800 medications. Go to Ira Bradley's room and click on **Vital Signs**.

3. Take a full set of vital signs and record them below. Then return to the Nurses' Station and open the EPR. Click on **Vital Signs** and chart your findings there.

   Blood pressure _____   Heart rate _____   Oxygen saturation _____

   Temperature _____   Respiratory rate _____   Pain rating _____

4. Was Ira Bradley wearing oxygen at the time you measured his O_2 saturation? How would knowledge about supplemental oxygen affect how you interpret this measurement?

5. Based on the vital sign results, what nursing action is indicated at this time?

6. What medications could you consider administering to Ira Bradley for pain? What information will you use to make this decision? *Hint:* Refer to textbook Chapter 12 or Lesson 6 of this workbook if needed for pain management information.

7. You have treated Ira Bradley's pain and have given him 30 minutes for it to take effect. Now you wish to conduct a shift nursing assessment. What precautions should you take while you are working with Ira Bradley to protect yourself from infection?

→ 8. Return to Ira Bradley's room, click on **Physical**, and observe the complete physical exam. Record your data below and place an asterisk next to any finding that is considered abnormal.

Assessment Area	Data Obtained
Head and Neck	
Chest/Upper Extremities	
Abdomen and Lower Extremities	

9. Based on the physical exam you observed, is there anything more you would like to assess? *Hint:* Data are missing from the examination of the upper and lower extremities.

→ It is time to give 0900 medications. While you are still in the patient's room, click on **Medications** and then on **Review Medications**. Compare the list of medications in the box with the list you reviewed earlier in the MAR. Now click on **Administer** to give Ira Bradley his medications.

10. Which medication is being given one hour later than it is scheduled on the MAR?

11. Using your clinical judgment, discuss whether or not this late dose is a serious issue and why.

12. How should the late dose in question 10 be documented on the MAR?

13. Should any further action be taken? Explain.

14. What two medications that were due at 0900 did not appear in the box while the nurse was administering medications?

15. Where would the topical medication (in question 14) most likely be kept?

16. What plausible reason could be there be for the medication in question 15 not being listed at this time?

17. What will you do to ensure that the other medication is available to administer?

➡ Now click on **Health History** and conduct a complete interview with Ira Bradley.

18. Record significant data from the health history interview for each of the following areas.

Health History Area	Ira Bradley's Data
Perception/Self-Concept	
Activity	
Sexuality/Reproduction	
Culture	
Nutrition/Metabolic	
Sleep/Rest	
Role/Relationship	
Health Perception	

Health History Area	Ira Bradley's Data
Elimination	
Cognitive/Perceptual	
Coping/Stress	
Value/Belief	

→ Return to the Supervisor's Office and sign in to work with Ira Bradley, this time on Thursday at 1100. Go to the Nurses' Station to find the location of the Health Team meeting for Ira Bradley. Go there, listen to the reports, and record significant data or concerns addressed by each member in question 19 (below and on the next page). Return to the patient's chart, click on **Health Team**, and read each member's written report. Record additional data in question 19.

19. What significant data or concerns were reported by each of the health team members?

Nurse case manager

Clinical nurse specialist

Social worker

 20. Review information about patient/family education and home care management for HIV and AIDS on pp. 1671–1672 of your textbook. Using all of the data you have acquired about Ira Bradley, briefly describe the similarities and differences between his case and the textbook discussion about patient education and community care for patients living with HIV/AIDS.

Problems of the Skin

 Reading Assignment: Problems of the Skin (Chapter 62)

Patients: Ira Bradley, Room 309

In this lesson you will focus on skin assessment and pressure ulcer prevention for Ira Bradley, a 43-year-old Caucasian male who is at risk for skin breakdown because of immobility.

Writing Activity

1. What is a pressure ulcer?

2. What population is most at risk for pressure ulcer development?

3. How does a patient's activity level affect the risk for developing a pressure ulcer?

4. Briefly describe the four pathophysiologic changes that occur in pressure ulcer development. *Hint:* Refer to Table 62-11 on p. 1974 in the textbook.

CD-ROM Activity

Go to the Supervisor's Office and sign in to work with Ira Bradley on Thursday at 0700. Go to the Nurses' Station and open his chart. Click on **History and Physical** and read the entire report, making note below of any information about mobility and skin condition.

Student Notes

Next, access Ira Bradley's EPR. Click on **Assessments** and review the entries for items that could relate to pressure ulcer development. Describe the data charted in the EPR for each of the entries listed below and on the next page.

5.	Monday 1600	Tuesday 1600	Wednesday 1600
Orientation			
Edema			

	Monday 1600	Tuesday 1600	Wednesday 1600
Motor strength/ sensation/mobility			
Skin assessment			

6. Does Ira Bradley's risk for pressure ulcer development increase or decrease from Monday to Wednesday based on documentation in the EPR? Explain.

 Next, click on **ADL** in the EPR. Note Ira Bradley's diet order (nutrition) and percentage of meals eaten (appetite) on Monday, Tuesday, and Wednesday at 1600.

7. What was Ira Bradley's nutritional data from Monday through Wednesday at 1600?

	Monday 1600	Tuesday 1600	Wednesday 1600
Nutrition			
Appetite			

8. Using all of the data you have gathered so far and the Braden Scale in Fig. 62-20 on pp. 1977–1978 of your textbook, determine scores for Ira Bradley's risk for pressure ulcer development from Monday through Wednesday. Refer to your answers to question 5 and question 7 to review individual data. If no specific data are available, use the lowest number to avoid underestimating his risk.

	Monday 1600	Tuesday 1600	Wednesday 1600
Sensory perception			
Moisture			
Activity			
Mobility			
Nutrition			
Friction and shear			
Total score			

9. Using the Braden Scale scores you calculated in question 8, identify how Ira Bradley's risk for pressure ulcer development has changed from Monday to Wednesday.

10. Does Ira Bradley have any skin breakdown at the present time according to the documentation in his chart? Does he have any other type of skin impairment?

11. Identify five skin care measures that can be used to prevent Ira Bradley from developing a pressure ulcer during his hospitalization. *Hint:* See Guidelines for Safe Practice on p. 1981 in the textbook.

12. Suggest six interventions related to mobility and activity to reduce Ira Bradley's risk for developing a pressure ulcer.

13. What general instructions would you include in patient and family education about reducing risk for pressure ulcer development after discharge?

Notes:

Notes:

Notes:

Notes:

Notes: